Hot Granny

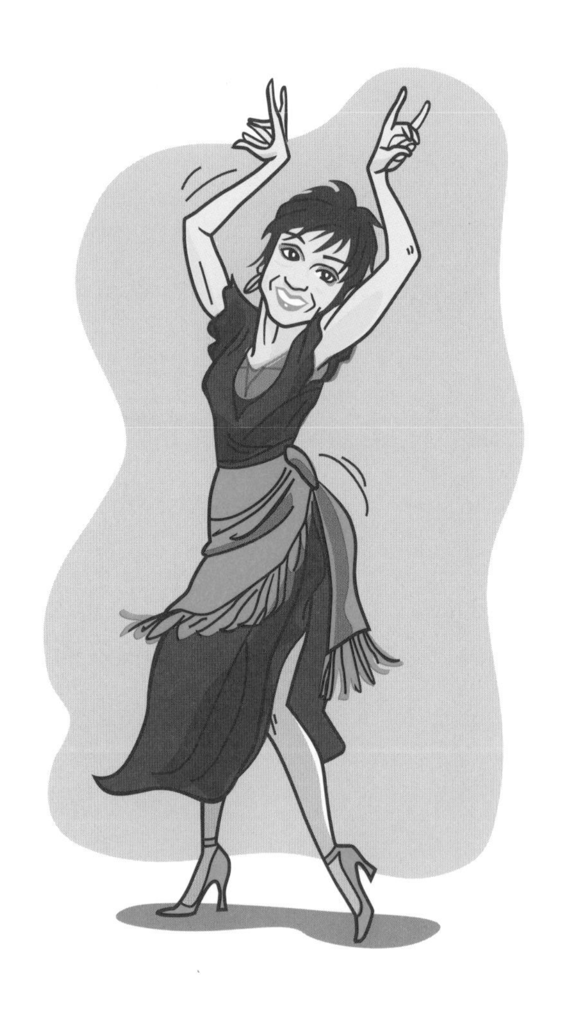

Hot Granny

FABULOUS AT 50, 60, AND BEYOND!

By Mel Walsh

Illustrations by Chuck Gonzales

CHRONICLE BOOKS
SAN FRANCISCO

To the Sister Listers . . .

over 100 Hot Grannies who inspired this book.

Library of Congress Cataloging-in-Publication Data available.

ISBN-10: 0-8118-5628-3
ISBN-13: 978-0-8118-5628-7

Manufactured in China

Designed by Amy Gregg

Distributed in Canada by Raincoast Books
9050 Shaughnessy Street
Vancouver, British Columbia V6P 6E5

10 9 8 7 6 5 4 3 2 1

Chronicle Books LLC
680 Second Street
San Francisco, California 94107

www.chroniclebooks.com

contents

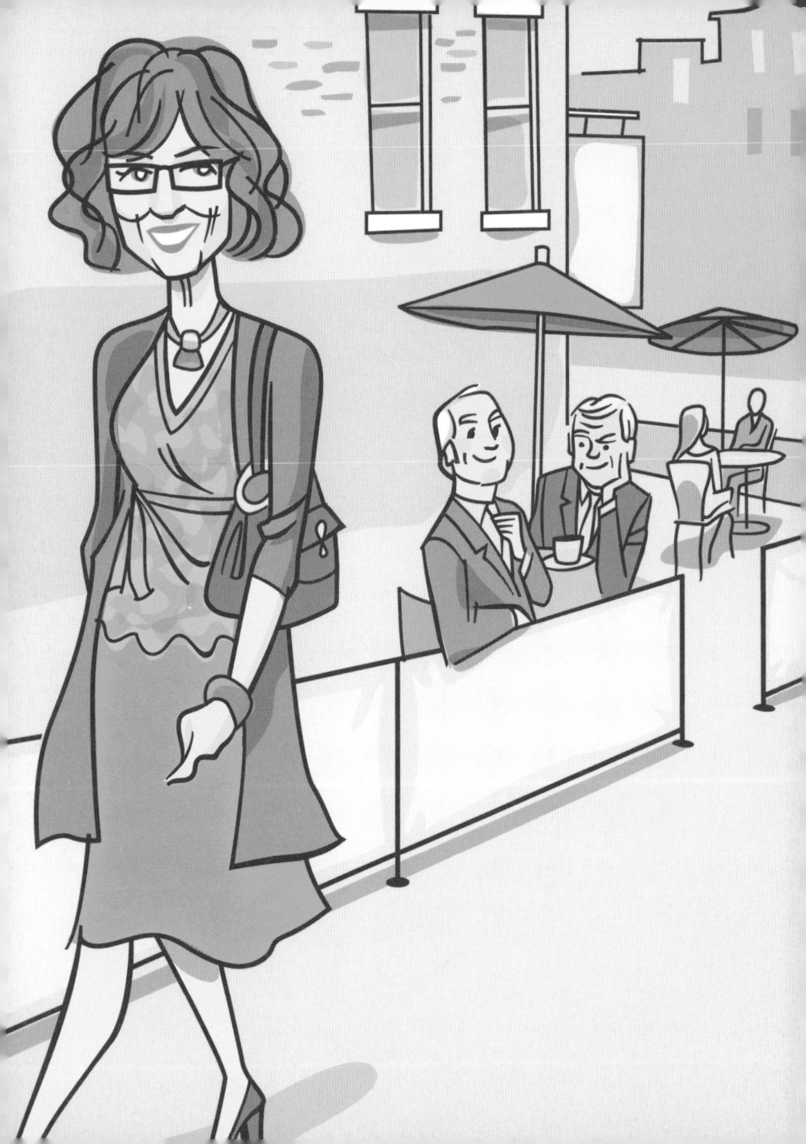

What's a Hot Granny? Basics for Beginners

× × × × ×

Hot.
Granny.

Yes, the two words go together. And we're not talking frequent-flasher hot—as in menopause—but "hot" as in "with-it and on top of the world."

And here's the really good part. If you are sailing past fifty, your ship has come in, because the world is finally catching on to the virtues of older women. That means older women are starting to see themselves as they are: bright, full of promise for the future, steadied by wisdom from the past. That's a very nice package at a very good time of life, a time of life reported by older people to be—ta dah!—*happy*.

Yes, happy. Happier than midlife. Happiest-since-childhood happy.

So, Hot Granny, look in the mirror, and say hi to your about-to-be-happy self. Whether you read this because you are a new grandmother, a single older woman, or just in need of a jump-start into the rest of your life, you will find life-tested advice here about the years ahead as well as inspiration to float you onward.

In fact, your life is a wonder of the modern world, a new thing under the sun.

Why? Because, whether you are single or married, whether a grandmother now or not, if you are over fifty and heading toward your silver age, you are both a lucky woman and a potential Hot Granny. One hundred years ago, the average woman was dead by her late forties. Out the door, toes up, *finito*. But today, in a history-making leap of good health and longevity, we older women have time—maybe thirty or forty extra years—to play, explore, laugh, love, learn, and develop our Hot Granny selves.

But, you may ask, what exactly is a Hot Granny? Does she have to score high on some babe scale? Must she be a fox?

Well, some women still ride high on the babe scale. Think of Goldie Hawn and Shirley MacLaine—both glam grannies. But a Hot Granny is way more than looks. Goldie and Shirley have certain spirits that make them Hot Grannies.

The Heart of a Hot Granny

Here's what it takes: a positive attitude, enthusiasm that's catchable, never giving up, courage, being totally yourself, loving others and loving what you do, keeping the brain in high gear, and being more involved with today and tomorrow than with yesterday. Those are the virtues that count. With those in your life, great things are possible for any older woman. You can look like a horse, walk like a chicken, have wrinkles like the side fissures of the Grand Canyon, and still be a Hot Granny.

That said—meaning it ain't just looks, babe, and beauty is only as deep as a surgeon's knife—a Hot

Granny who respects herself will still try to be her best self. She'll pay some attention to her looks, if only so she won't scare people at the mall. And if she's single and thinking of doubling, she may give her looks more than a second thought. A Hot Granny will also pay attention to her physical self, so she won't poop out at sixty or seventy and begin asking that heartbreaking question: "Whatever became of me?"

And because a Hot Granny has a heart, she won't give up on her hopes of love ever after. And because she has a body designed for loving, she won't give up on pleasure, either.

In my book, a Hot Granny isn't even required to have a grandchild. She just has to care what happens to the next generation. Any woman who cares qualifies. And that's every older woman I know. We care. It's our lifetime specialty—and we're not giving up on it now.

What's at the Heart of This Book?

To help you find your path through the World of Older, this book specifically offers real-world advice about relationships with friends, lovers, and mates. Take only what suits your life as an older woman. You'll also

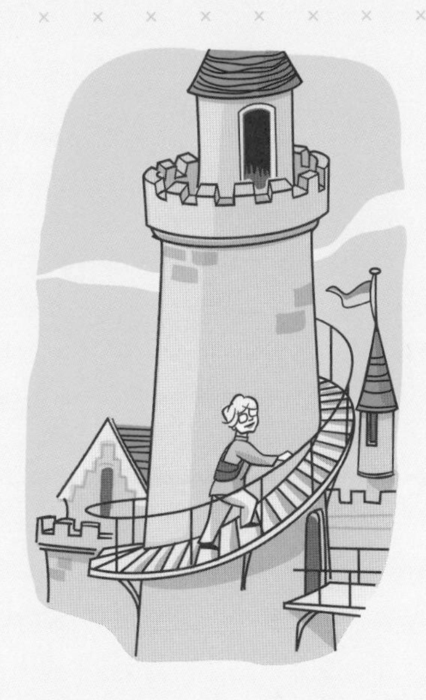

find information on how to keep yourself in shape so you can do the things you dreamed about when you were younger. (You can't climb to the top of that castle in Scotland unless your legs and lungs are in good shape.) Looking good is on the menu here, and family matters are in the spotlight, too: how to enjoy small people, the little rug puppies of our lives, and also how to enjoy the bigger ones, such as the older husband or the silver-haired lover. Hot Granny's dreams for her life are encouraged in detail—whether those dreams involve travel, creativity, education, or new pursuits of long-held ambitions. So, whether you are an actual grandmother, whether you are fifty or seventy, there is something here for you.

As for me, your guide to Hot Grannydom, I am a nonfiction author and columnist, a gerontologist, and the host of a radio show for older adults, *Second Wind*. On the Web, I live at www.melwalsh.com.

On the family side, I am a grandmother of twelve and recently remarried—yes, later-life love—to a Hot Grandpa called Mac, who keeps telling me he's going to retire. But the fact is, he loves the law so much, he doesn't want to leave it. Nor should he, for a Hot Grandpa needs to play by the same rules as a Hot Granny—stay passionate about what you do.

I'm telling you about my life in this introduction, not because I think I am so wonderful, but because I think the opportunities for older women in the twenty-first century are more than wonderful. For instance, I took the Graduate Record Examination in my sixties—and then went to graduate school to study gerontology, the science of older people. Later, to tell others about growing more vital while aging well, I learned how to broadcast and engineer a radio show. Imagine a show with jazz and gerontology, vintage music, and contemporary talk about life after fifty. Then, to tell even more people about the good life after fifty, I began a newspaper column.

So, there are many doors for a Hot Granny to open as she looks beyond her kids—now grown—and beyond her job—perhaps retired from—toward a new life. These challenges will keep the brain from congealing like day-old oatmeal.

Sure, some of it is scary, but goofing is how people of all ages learn. Which all goes to show you that it's progress, not perfection, that we're after here.

So, go for it, Hot Granny. Catch your second wind. Follow your path.

But make it your own path. As the saying on my fridge door goes, "Be who you is, because if you is who you ain't, you ain't who you is."

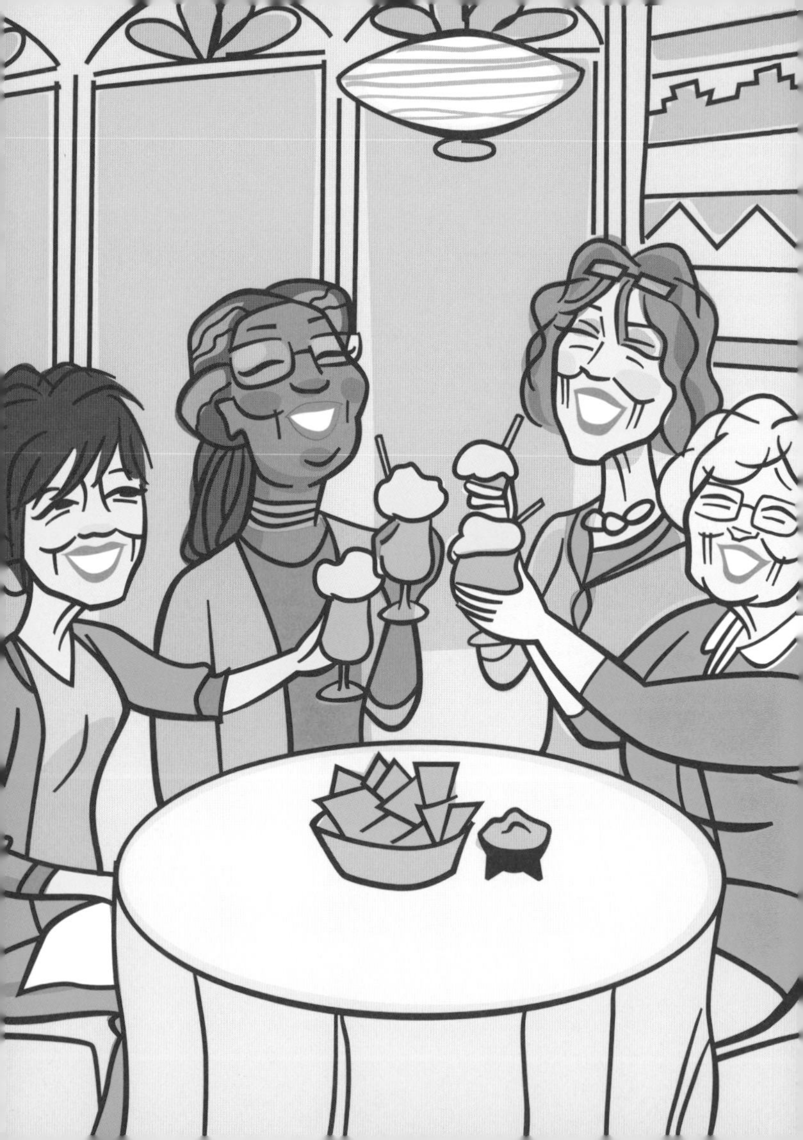

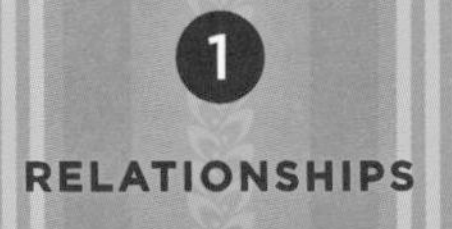

Hot Granny and the Girlfriends

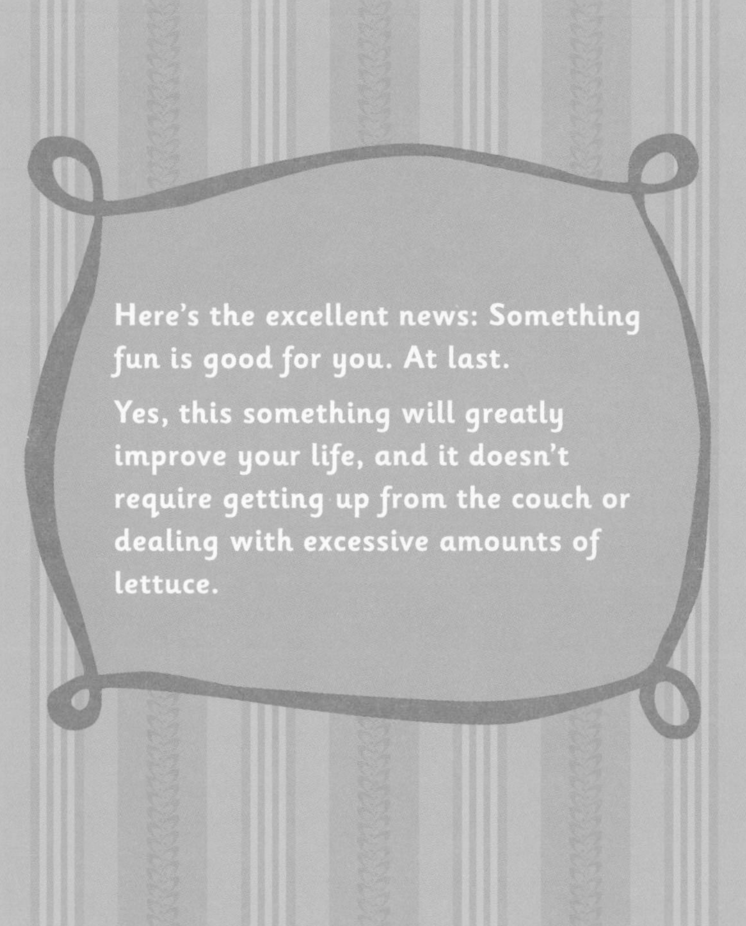

Here's the excellent news: Something fun is good for you. At last.

Yes, this something will greatly improve your life, and it doesn't require getting up from the couch or dealing with excessive amounts of lettuce.

As you have heard and heard until your ears go numb, experts tell us to do three things for our well-being.

1. **EXERCISE FORTY-FIVE MINUTES A DAY.**
   (IN YOUR DREAMS.)

2. **EAT FIVE TO NINE SERVINGS OF FRUITS AND VEGETABLES A DAY.**
   (HOW DO WE PULL THIS ONE OFF?)

3. **GIGGLE WITH THE GIRLFRIENDS.**
   (NOW YOU'RE TALKING.)

Seriously, friends are a proven prescription for emotional health: Take one girlfriend and call her in the morning. Gerontologists call this "socialization," but women call it fun. Party hearty with the sisters. Go gigglebritches with another gal. Laugh so hard you wet your pants—these are the things friendship dreams are made of.

And here's the even better news: as females, we are the naturally talented sex when it comes to making friends. Males form alliances around work, and other than that, many settle for a lone-cowhand life—the tough, self-sufficient guy riding off into the sunset.

Sure, some socially intelligent guys keep up the childhood and school connections and also hang out with sports and hobby buddies, and a wise Hot Granny encourages this in her man, though it may mean golf or football widowhood now and then. But too many older men have just one main friend: their wives. That can exert a lot of pressure on a Hot Granny, especially when her man is retired and just hanging around the kitchen. (Don't feed him, or he'll never leave.)

Now, on the other hand, you don't hear about lone cowgirls. In general, women aren't wired that way. Lucky for us.

Friends in Later Life

But isn't it the truth that friends were easier to get way back when? School recess was an excellent place to harvest girlfriends. Then, when we grew up, the neighborhood, the workplace, the circle of other parents—all these were easy places to find buddies.

But life after fifty may present a few challenges. Example: You may leave your friends. Yes, you. If you move to another town in retirement, you may know few people and will have to polish up your friendship skills, including how to walk up to strangers and start a conversation, how to suggest future get-togethers, and how to maintain the fun and forward momentum of a friendship. All these things we learned in kindergarten and can recapture again. Yes, there may be rejection or evident disinterest, but don't take it personally.

Why? Well, the people you approach may already have developed friendship networks and enjoy extensive armies of relatives. They can't squeeze in one more person—unless it's Paul Newman or Robert Redford. The date books are full, and you're coming in late to their party.

Then, too, there's another complication to friendship after fifty: Our best friends may leave us—either to live out their own retirement dreams in a different area or to move on to Heavenly Acres. This is a fact of life, but people who love people will find new compatibles. Not that any special friend can be replaced, but the gap left by that friend can be filled with another just as special in a different way.

The world is full of Hot Grannies, and our task is to find them.

Getting Fussy About Friends

Something else is going on when it comes to later-life friendships—something gerontologists call "social selectivity." That means, as we grow older, we don't waste our time on people we don't like because we know in our bones we don't have forever on this planet. Time is short, and why waste it on people we hate?

Increasingly, as we grow older, we don't. Which is not to say we are rude to people, just that we no longer say yes when an Ultra-Bitch suggests lunch. Hot Grannies only lunch with ladies.

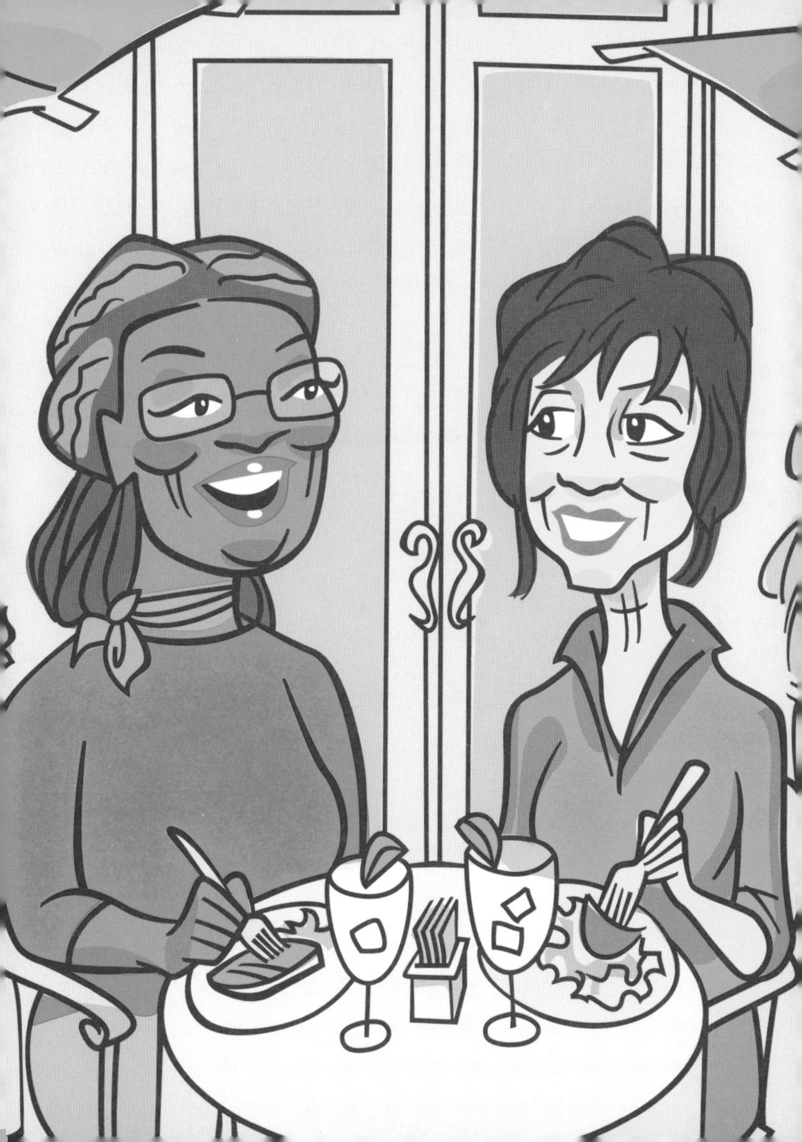

Finding Girlfriends After Fifty

THE POOL OF AVAILABLE GIRLFRIENDS MAY SHRINK AS A HOT GRANNY GROWS OLDER, ESPECIALLY IF SHE RETIRES FROM THE WORKPLACE. SO HOW DO HOT GRANNIES FIND MORE FRIENDS?

- Go back and re-find old friends you've lost touch with over the years. Internet search engines such as www.google.com are your own personal detective agency. Enter several versions of your buddy's name: Jane Nasmith Plover, Mrs. John Plover, Jane Nasmith. Write inquiries to alum magazines. Go to class reunions. Join any class bulletin boards on the Internet.
- Go with your passion for doing good in the world. Volunteer for something you believe in—whether it's animal rescue, preventing child abuse, or delivering meals to the homebound. You should discover at least one friend who feels the way you do about the world.
- Join a group with similar beliefs and interests. This could be a political party at the local level, a church, or a civic or arts organization. Go to the meetings. Donate time and expertise.

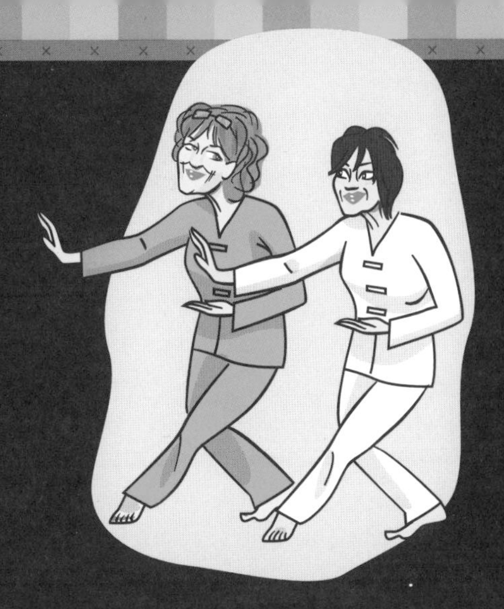

- Meet your girlfriends' girlfriends. But be thoughtful, and don't exclude the first friend from future social occasions. That's behaving like a bad third-grader.
- Take courses. Go back to school. Here's where you found friends before. School still works.
- Join fitness groups. Pilates, yoga, tai chi, jazz dance, water aerobics—they all attract like-minded women.
- Talk to neighbors. They are probably not all ax murderers.
- Talk to strange women on airplanes. (One of them introduced me to my husband.)

Why Women Pals Grow More and More Important

Girlfriends were essential when you wanted to play double-Dutch jump rope—probably our first cooperative adventure as females—and if you think you needed gal pals then, wait until you are an experienced Hot Granny.

Here's why smart Hot Grannies put time and love into friendships: They finally have the time. Kids are gone; workplace involvement has probably diminished. There is now space on the calendar for lunch, coffee, dinner, giggles, movie nights, wine bars, and shopping. This is one great reward for growing older: having time for friends.

Older women know this is the time of life to pay special attention to friends. When women retire, there are no more workplace buddies and social celebrations at the office. If women are widowed, they may need ears to listen and hands to help them through their grief and redirect their social interests.

All older women could use a little caretaking after years of giving it to others. Translate *caretaking* into chicken soup appearing at a sickroom door, mail and newspapers taken care of when someone's away, rides to auto repair shops or medical appointments, or

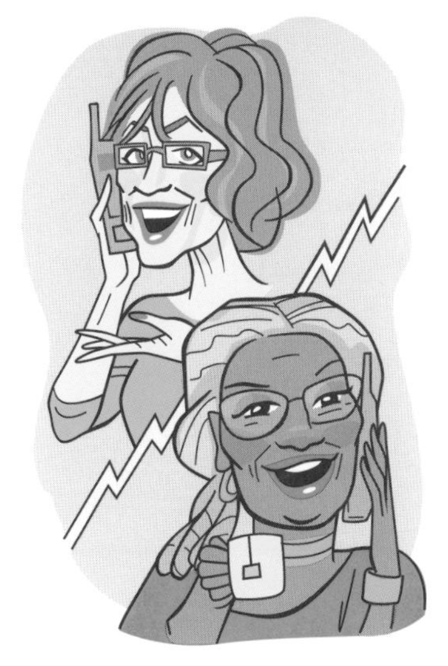

designated night driving for night-blind friends. And any Hot Granny worth the title will want to give as well as receive these kindnesses.

Hot Grannies are the gender that inherits the planet. Men die several years before their female age peers. Big shortage of men. So, who are we going to be friends with? Our kids have their own lives. Girlfriends are the answer. Blessed be the sisters.

Hot Grannies who surround themselves with friends will be better off. Period. The research says friends are crucial to well-being in later life, so don't go into a cave as an older woman. Stay out in the world with the girls. And give them a copy of this book to celebrate the friendship.

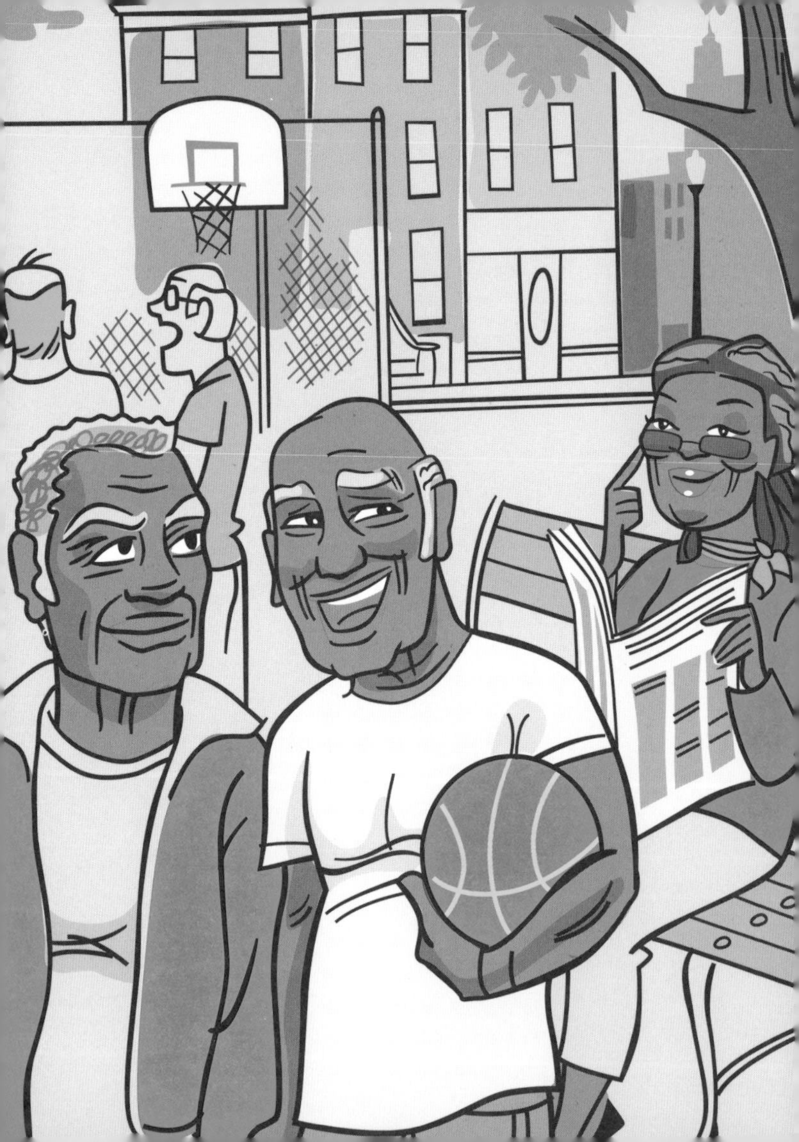

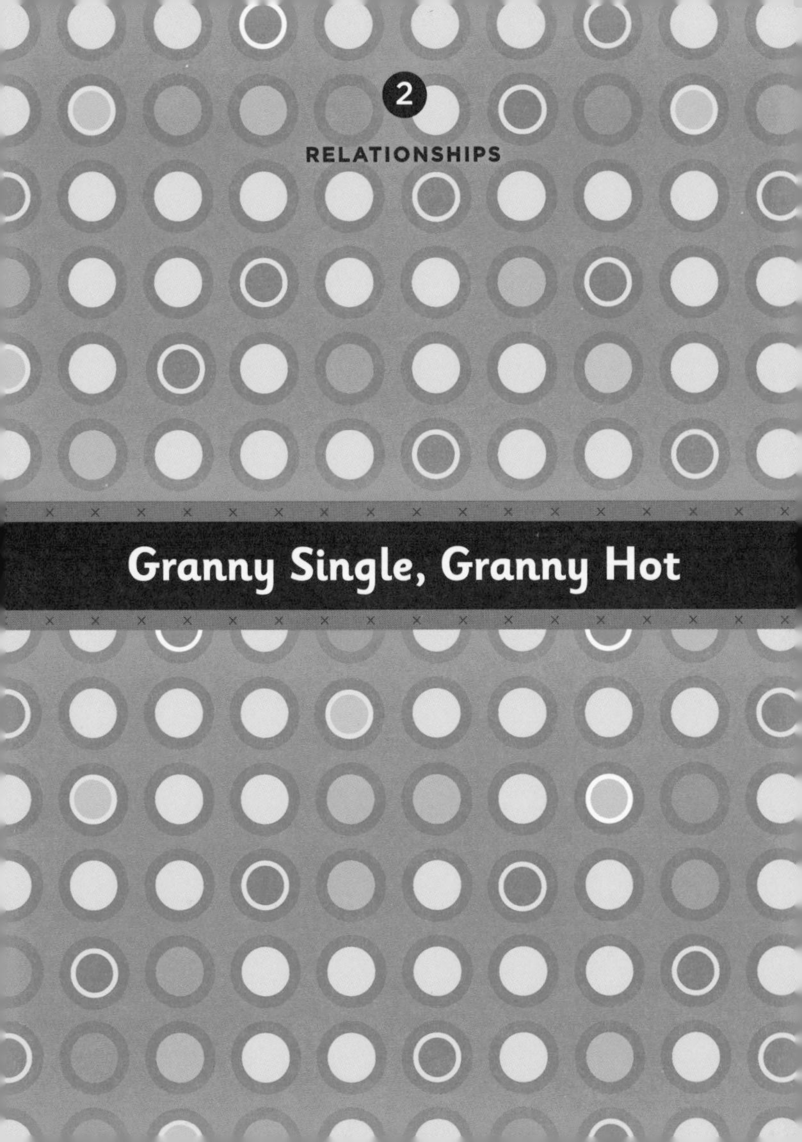

2

RELATIONSHIPS

Granny Single, Granny Hot

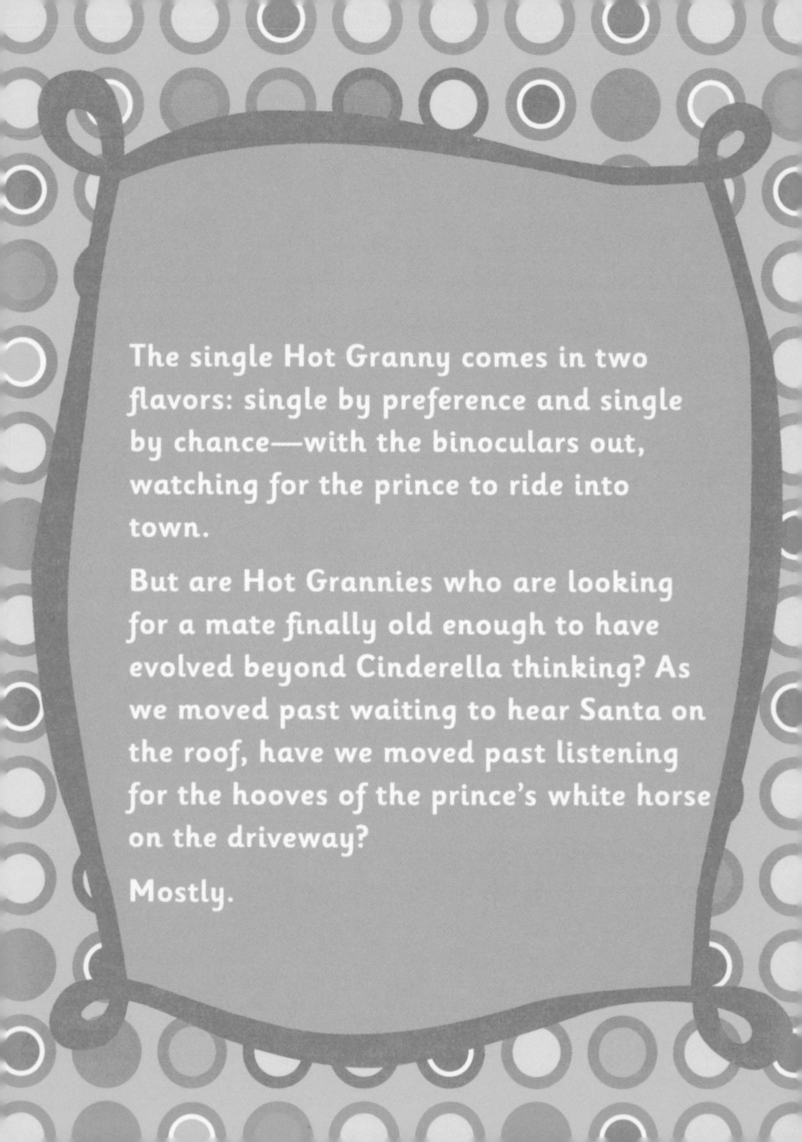

The single Hot Granny comes in two flavors: single by preference and single by chance—with the binoculars out, watching for the prince to ride into town.

But are Hot Grannies who are looking for a mate finally old enough to have evolved beyond Cinderella thinking? As we moved past waiting to hear Santa on the roof, have we moved past listening for the hooves of the prince's white horse on the driveway?

Mostly.

In our sane hours, we realize that no prince is coming to town, but that there are perfectly nice men already there, some of them just as flawed and imperfect as those of us who seek them. And that is the beginning of wisdom for the single Hot Granny looking for a mate. Seek not beyond what you yourself offer. I figure that if I am about 75 percent OK and 25 percent a pain in the posterior—the usual human mix—I probably should look for a man who registers about the same on the life-partner scale.

Now, if a Hot Granny wants to drive herself to drink and despair, she sets her sights on perfection. Do this and expect to spend your nights in bed alone with an empty pizza box for company.

Manicures may be perfect. Men are not.

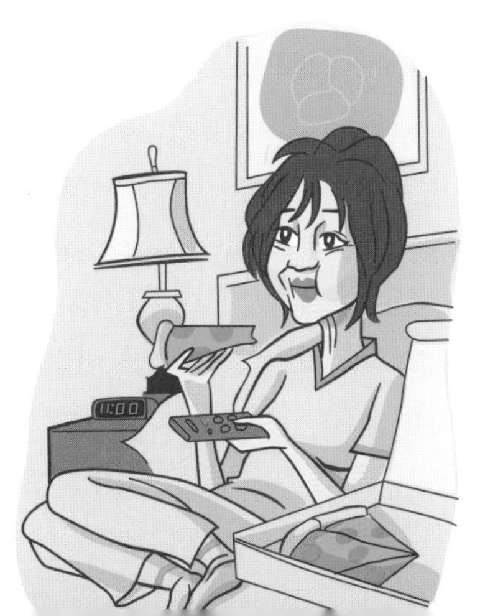

Are All the Good Ones Taken?

If all the good men are taken, why do the wedding pages of the *New York Times* regularly report marriages of people who find each other later in life? All the good ones are not taken. But like musical chairs, there are more people than landing spots. As noted, men have an unfortunate habit of dying younger than women.

That means, as we get older, there are more women, fewer men. Whoa! More competition. But if you want to polish and shine up the human being that is you, Hot Granny, and become an even hotter granny, then don't miss the two chapters in the next section, "Self."

Where to Find the Single Male

The single men are out there, but how do Hot Grannies find them?

Try: The vast resources of other women. They know men. They have address books and memories. Their cousins, their coworkers, and even their rejects may be just what would interest you. And you don't have to already know all these helpful women. Unless a stranger is conversing with an imaginary friend, talk to her. As I noted earlier, I met my husband by talking to a woman sitting next to me on a plane. Women enjoy making matches, so float along on this kindness. Return it when you can.

Try: Getting out into the world of organizations. You may not be a joiner, but get your Hot Granny self over to the sign-up sheet at some organization you are truly interested in. I know two women who met fabulous husbands at political fund-raisers. Or get a sports car and join a car club. If anything has wheels, there's always a club with men in it. Don't forget Rotary, Elks, and other formerly all-male clubs. They still have many men as members. Volunteering also makes sense. Work at soup kitchens, deliver meals-on-wheels, and collect clothes for the dispossessed.

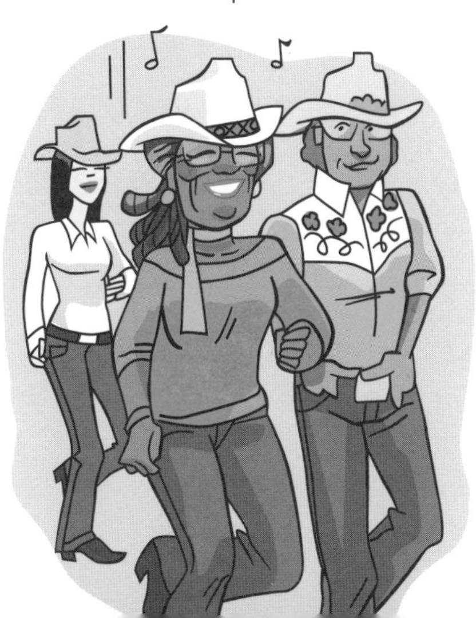

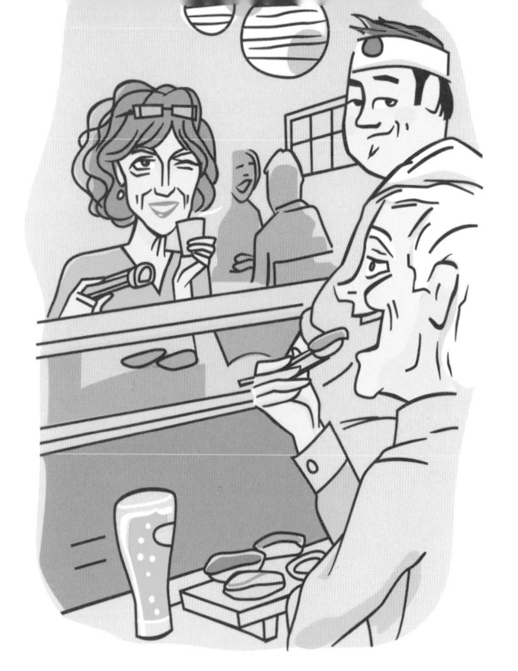

Try: Taking a class. If you like the idea of country streams plus peace and quiet, take a fly-fishing class. (Only worm-free fishing for a Hot Granny.) Or go to a line-dancing class. Take *taiko* drumming lessons. Even watercolor classes will work. Yes, they may be all-woman classes, but see the first item in this section.

Try: Travel. Take a cruise. Go someplace, anyplace. Go to the theater and concerts while you're there. Talk to people on the road. Talk to people in museums—a very good place to meet people. If you don't like to eat alone, try sushi bars and restaurants with communal breakfast bars.

Try: Recovery organizations. If you have had a struggle with substance abuse, find an organization that encourages sobriety. I have a single friend who travels extensively, serene in the knowledge that almost anywhere she goes, she will be welcomed by fellow AA members—all of whom have a similar idea about how to have a good time.

Try: Getting active. Take out a gym membership, and use it. Hike with the Sierra Singles. Join a biking club.

Try: The performing arts. Join a theater group, a choir, anything musical.

Try: The Internet. The Net is an adventure in cyberspace, but watch your back and know that many men who advertise for company already have it—they're married.

Dating in the Mellow Years

Here's the first fact. If you haven't dated in a while, or even if you have, first dates as an older woman are just as nerve-wracking as they were when you were sixteen. Mellow years, same fears. Even the questions are the same:

- WHAT IF YOU HATE EACH OTHER?
- WHAT IF YOU REALLY LIKE HIM AND HE DOESN'T LIKE YOU?
- WHAT IF HE LIKES YOU AND YOU HATE HIM?
- SHOULD YOU ______ ON THE FIRST DATE?

But some concerns are different:

- YOU WILL NO LONGER WASTE TIME ON JERKS.
- YOU WILL SURVIVE IF HE DOESN'T LIKE YOU.
- YOU NOW KNOW HOW TO GRACEFULLY DISENGAGE IF YOU WANT TO.
- YOU CAN FINALLY TRUST YOURSELF TO DECIDE WHAT YOU WANT TO DO ON A FIRST DATE.

Of course, today you are also wise enough to start small—a coffee date—and in public—a coffeehouse—and to check the smoking, drinking, and drug habits that might peek out at first acquaintance. Money issues can arise even on first dates, and if he asks you to split the check for lattes, that's the sign of a miser.

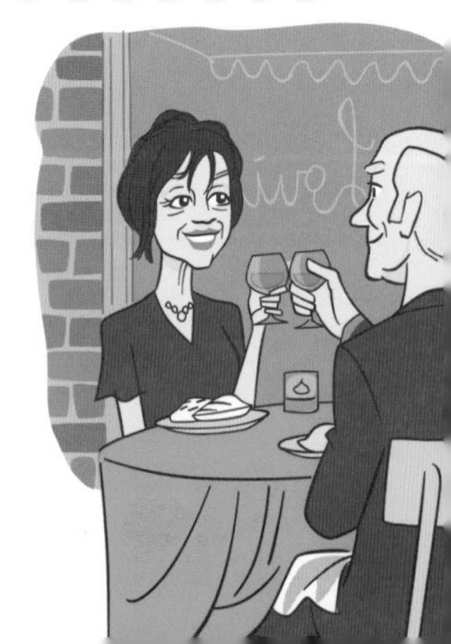

Internet Adventures

Dating sites on the Internet have proliferated like horny bunnies. Each site may have different rules: photos required or not; membership fee or not. But all will ask you to say something about yourself.

If you have trouble tooting your own horn, you can ask a friend to help you with the write-up. Veterans of cyberdating suggest getting a book to learn how to write an appealing profile, take a good photograph, and discover ways to protect your personal privacy, such as www.myprivateline.com, a service that provides a toll-free number that can be forwarded to your real home phone or cell number. That's so you don't have to give out your home phone right away (or ever).

If you do decide to cyberdate, wear a well-tailored rhino hide. Older women can get bruised by the reality that some men are only after younger game. And the going standards used to evaluate women are usually not related to character, kindness, or experience—but related to cuteness, bust size, and layability. So, cyberdater, beware. And if your ego starts shrinking into a dry dustball because of rejections, stop the Internet action and get back to flesh-and-blood introductions.

If you are about to date someone you met on the Internet, be smart: Call him first to talk before you

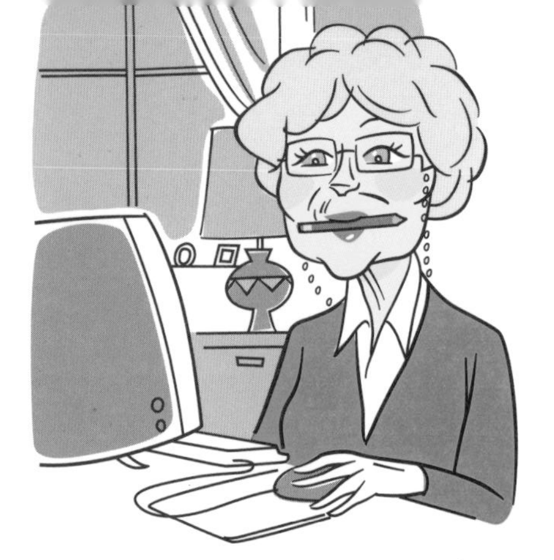

meet, meet in a public place for a short date, tell a friend where you are going and with whom, keep the date short and the drinking (if any) very moderate, have an exit strategy, and let it be known beforehand. Example: "I'll need to get back to the office (or off to gym class)." Ask direct questions about his marital status, and certainly be on your guard if you can only call him at his office in the future. And don't go off with him in his car on the first date.

Yes, you probably know all this by now, but sometimes safety issues are hard to remember when a man is a charming single and the drinks are delightful doubles.

And if you eventually become intimate with anyone, remember condoms. Neither of you needs a problem disease as a later-life companion.

More Little Realities

Issues that are obvious on any first date will be more obvious later on. My husband spent our first dinner date staring at my chest. I asked him if he planned on doing that all night or if he would try focusing on another spot—like my eyes. He did, but even today, he nearly drives off the pavement when any well-endowed woman jogs on the side of the road. So, don't expect a guy to change. Expect him to relax over time, but not to change.

And don't be discouraged if a man's family members don't jump on your bandwagon right away. They may have seen him get hurt. Also, later in life, some adult kids fear that Dad may leave it all to some upstart wife. If you get that far in a relationship, you can defuse fears by doing the right thing—which in my book is leaving his money to his kids, leaving your money to yours, and leaving each other the survivor's right to live off the interest. But, of course, different strokes prevail here. Consult a lawyer to prevent inheritance problems. Also, be aware how you both will do as a couple when it comes to Social Security income—married versus unmarried. Government policy still promotes Hot Grannies living in sin.

Sex—Again and Still

Why are people uncomfortable at the thought of older people making love? The fact is, older people have it all over younger people.

Older lovers don't get into bed and into relationships just because they're curious. They already know the physical geography, the lay of the lay.

Older people don't act like rabbits on speed. They understand the word *slow*.

Older people don't have to worry about pregnancy or the time of the month. A diaphragm is now something you breathe with.

Older people know they don't have to pretend they love the person next to them. Real love is highly preferable, of course, but not required when in the investigative stage of dating.

Older lovers know more techniques, cuddling among them. They also have their own simple sex code—call it the Gero-Sutra—and it does not necessarily involve putting your legs up over your head. It may sometimes even involve the restful positions promoted by missionaries.

Older people have a sense of humor in bed—an underrated virtue in early romantic life, essential later on.

Single Hot Grannies don't worry if a guy will respect them in the morning. They wonder if they will respect the guy in the morning.

For tips on the physical side of love, see chapter 5, "The Very Warm Granny and Her Mate."

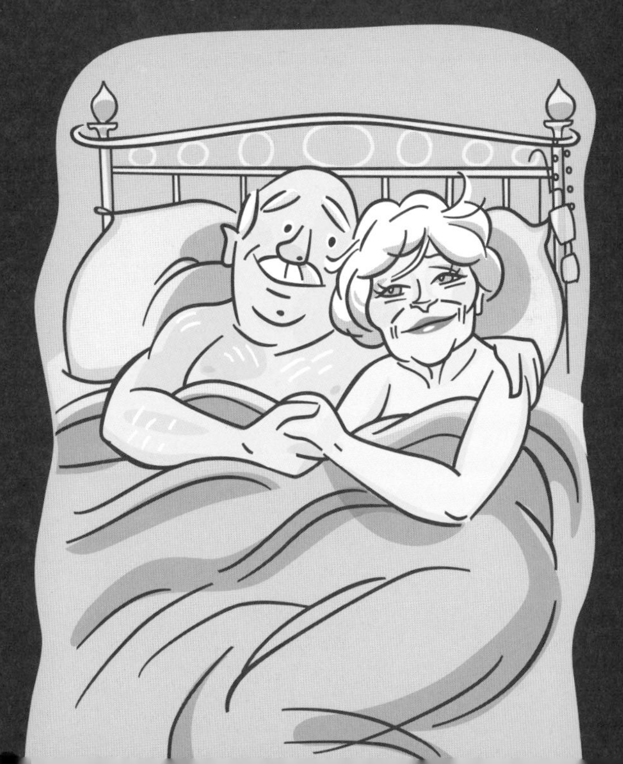

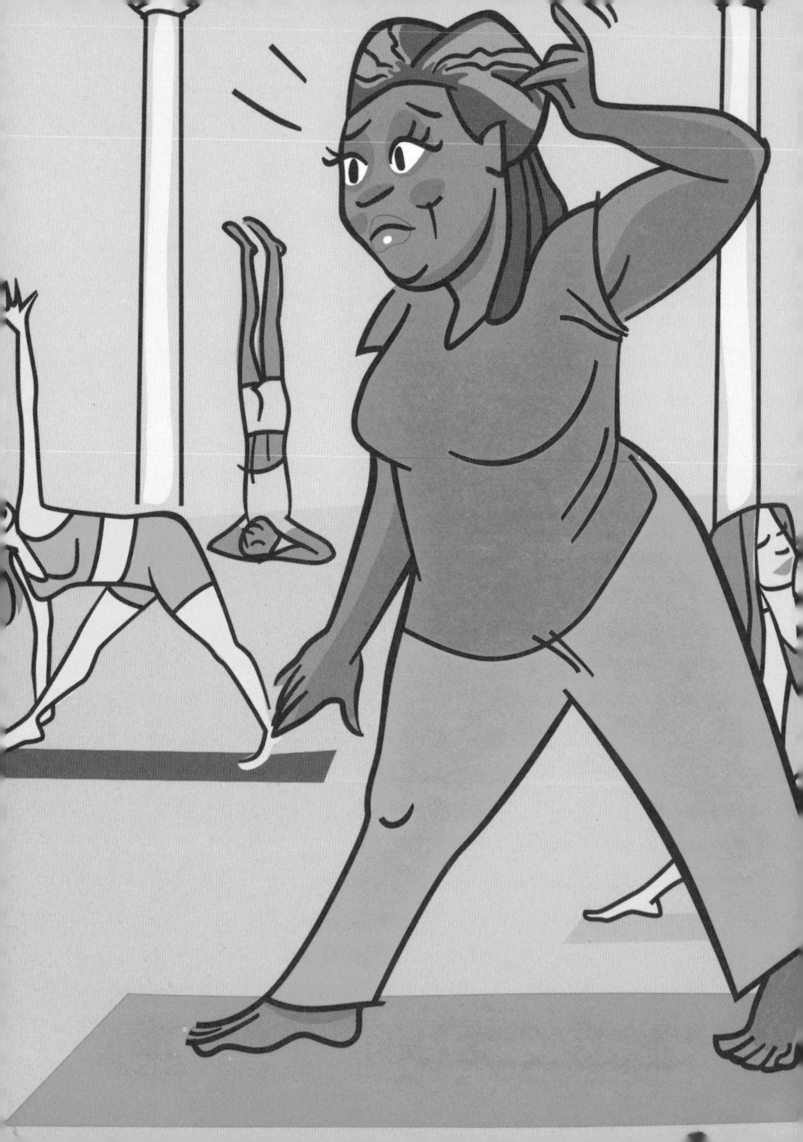

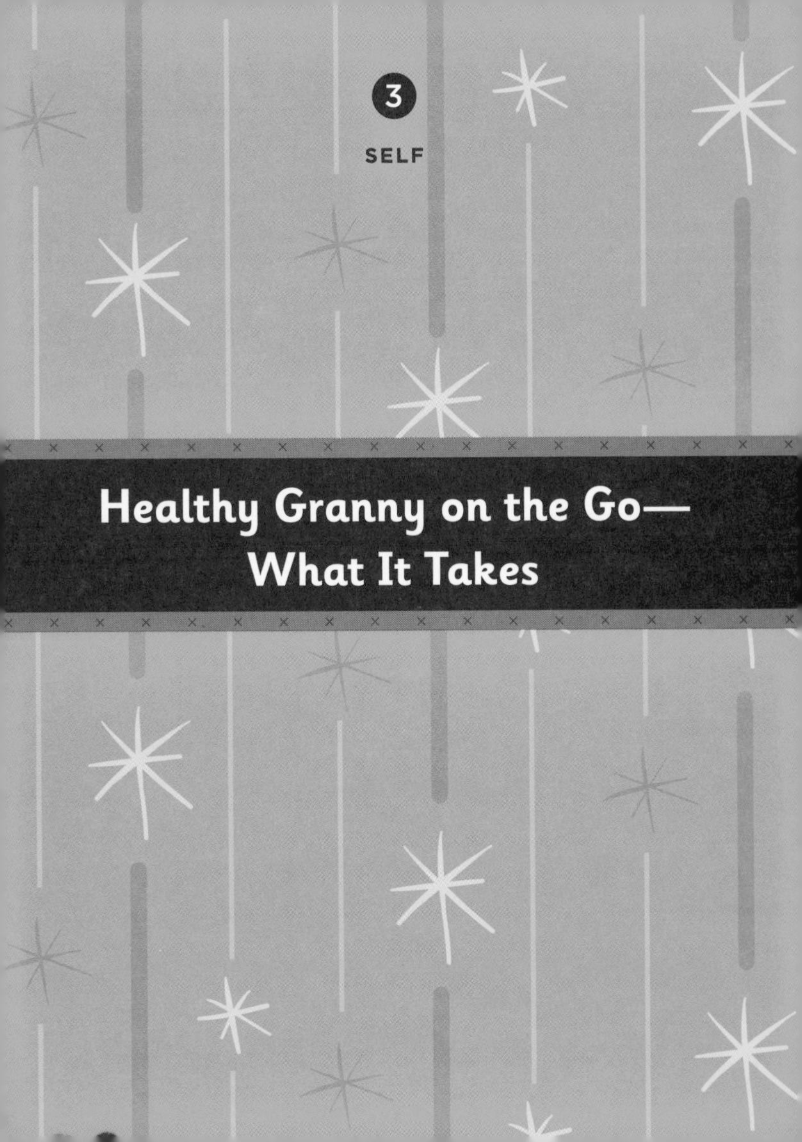

3

SELF

Healthy Granny on the Go—What It Takes

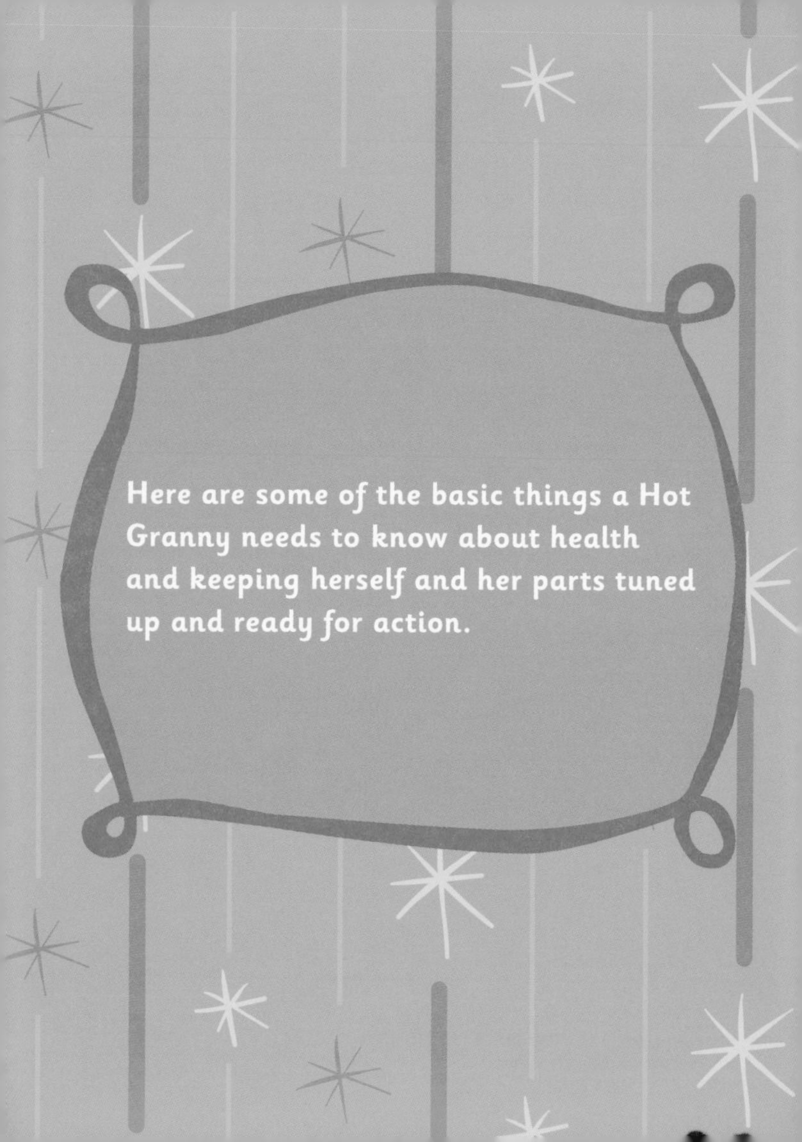

Here are some of the basic things a Hot Granny needs to know about health and keeping herself and her parts tuned up and ready for action.

The Body

Move your bottom off the couch. The rest of you must go along too. Swing your moving parts around almost every day for as long as it takes to watch a half-hour TV show. Exercising in front of the TV set is a painless way to tuck aerobic exercise into your life. These motions are supposed to be weight-bearing exercise. (Many of us have the weight all ready to go and have been bearing it for quite a while.)

Also, lift a few weights while you're at it. When dancing in front of the TV set, you can lift cans of beans up and down—silly, but it works—or use real weights, sold in any sports department. Tell yourself that strength is an asset as you go into a time of life when unexercised women may totter toward frailty.

Flexibility is also an asset as we move along in life, and it can be maintained or regained by stretching exercises and yoga. If you think flexibility is not important, look at older people whose body motions are as rigid as puppets. Women who want to look younger by erasing their wrinkles would be wise to also look at erasing stiffness in their bodies. Supple is young. Inflexible is not.

The Diet

Eat fruits, veggies, and whole grains, as well as soap-sized helpings of protein that are not floating in fat. Sugar and white flour are frowned upon, but I figure those rules don't count if you are eating pastries in Paris.

Seriously, you may have cooked for others your whole life and had to consider their dietary prejudices when making menus. But now you can concentrate more on what you want to eat that's healthy. Suggestion: A Mediterranean diet seems to suit the mind-set of many women. It's easy to imagine oneself in Tuscany—living in a villa, sitting under the olive trees, having a glass of wine, and enjoying foods *Italiano*. Nutritionists agree with this lifestyle, and for the clueless cook, there are many cookbooks and TV shows that tell what to buy and how to prepare it when you want to go Mediterranean.

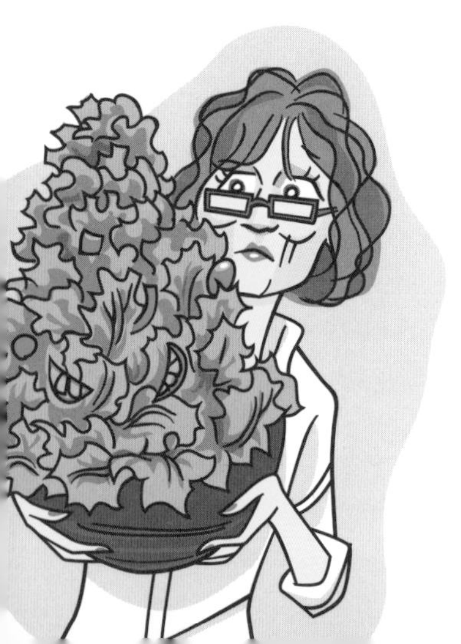

The Rest of It

Don't smoke or overdrink. Don't do street drugs or begin begging various docs for just another prescription of that painkiller that Donny lent you after his operation.

Do have a glass of red wine a day—it's supposedly good for the circulatory system, but that's only if you don't have trouble with alcohol or are not about to drive. Yes, most people can legally drive in the United States with only one drink in the system, but the older you are, the harder it may be to drive well, especially at night. It's not wise to add alcohol to the mix of things that make night driving somewhat exciting for older people: restricted vision, slower reaction times, more and faster traffic every year, new roads and freeways, and bright oncoming halogen headlights. On the other hand, a nice little Pinot Noir at home may do good things to your blood vessels and frame of mind.

If you stay away from the rear of diesel trucks, that will be good. Also, don't spray yourself with pesticides if you can help it.

Be your own watchdog when it comes to medical care. Charts get mixed up, prescriptions clash, and drugs are too often used to clear up symptoms that a lifestyle change could address more cheaply and with no side effects. Older Americans are in danger of becoming the designated drug takers of the country. Think twice before you go down the heavily medicated road without considering alternatives. Some older adults take ten to twelve drugs daily, get them mixed up, and take the wrong dosage. Use a pill-dispensing box to keep your meds straight and keep you out of the ER.

To keep yourself on the go, don't hesitate to replace hips and knees if they no longer serve well. Find a top surgeon in a top hospital, someone who often performs the specific operation that's going to get you on the dance floor again.

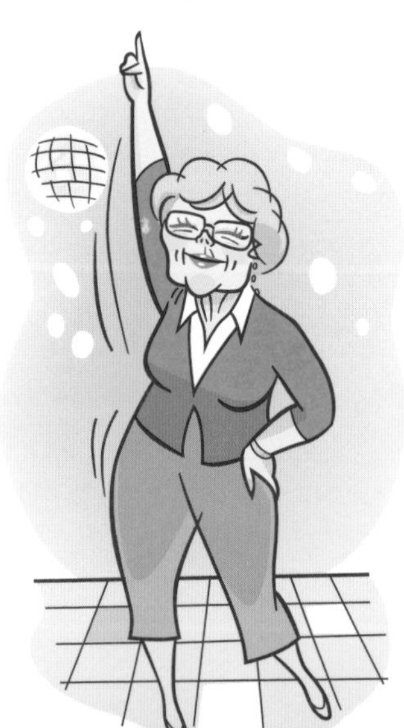

Replacing Parts: Medical Solutions to Hobbles and Squints

HOBBLES

Some older women don't like to think about going into the operating room for body work. Doesn't it mean you're old? Well, you're not, but your bones may be getting on. Seriously, skeletons can wear out—hips and knees in particular—and to get around in the years ahead and move your way into a healthy lifestyle, you do need a body that works and doesn't hurt.

Bone-on-bone pain when a hip needs help is enough to wake you up at night with the howling yowlies. And some women could write a book: *When Bad Knees Happen to Good People*. So, if your hips and knees need attention, do the following so you can get back to dancing:

Get over the fear of surgery by reading the stats. The vast majority of people who have had these operations are immensely satisfied, restored to function, and out of pain.

Go to your family doc. Get a beginning diagnosis and a referral to an orthopedist. Check around for names on your own, too. Ask about the very best and most experienced orthopedic surgeons in your wide

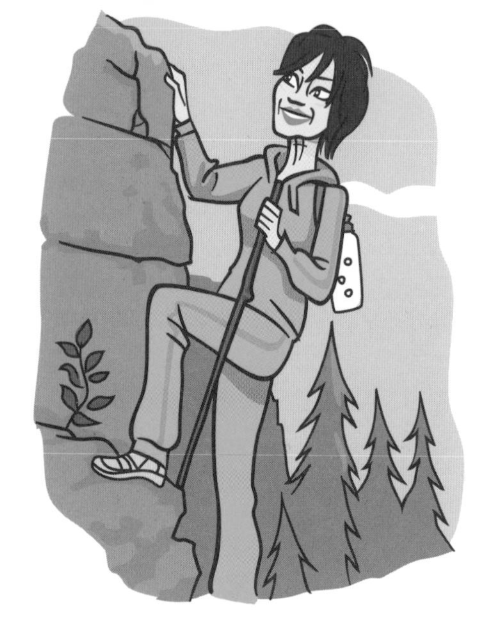

area. Don't stint on this research. Ask nurses: they know the skinny.

If you live in Burgersville and neither the doc nor the hospital has much experience with the operation you are going to have, get the heck out of Burgersville. Experience, although not everything, is very, very important when choosing a surgeon, a hospital, and the nursing care that goes with that hospital.

Post-op pain control is good nowadays, and physical therapy will get you on your feet in days. Do your boring therapy exercises, and you will be back to the dance floor and the hiking trail fast.

SQUINTS

The eyes of a Hot Granny may also need attention as she moves past fifty and sixty. If you've already "done" middle age, you know how growing older can change vision. You may be using reading glasses right now. Cute ones, of course.

Now, as we grow older, cataracts are the most common eye problem that can benefit from surgical treatment. More than twenty million Americans have this clouding of the lens, which, in surgery, is removed and replaced with a clear lens. No big deal to have done—no pain, much gain—and Hot Granny's vision is likely to be greatly improved . . . the better for night driving to exciting places, m'dear.

Some risk factors for cataracts are smoking, sun exposure, nearsightedness, and the use of steroids—whether those steroids are inhaled, put on the skin, or swallowed. The higher the dose, the higher the risk of cataracts.

But how do you know when Hot Granny's lenses are going south? Symptoms to look for: glare and halos around lights; blurred, cloudy, or fuzzy vision; frequent changes in eyeglass prescriptions; and poor night vision. There's also a slight yellowing of everything in the field of vision, and when you do have the surgery done, it can seem as though the world, which used to look like an old varnished painting, is now tinged with blue. Bright blue skies again. Very nice.

Don't be afraid to have cataract surgery. Again, get the best, most experienced surgeon. For more info about the older eye, visit www.agingeye.net.

Last, a tip about seeing better when driving on your granny-on-the-go rounds: Some older people see much better driving when they wear glasses with yellow lenses. A yellow lens ups the contrast; the change in visual sharpness can be dramatic.

So, stay healthy, and stay in motion. Do everything medically sensible to shore up any body parts showing signs of disobedience. Any Hot Granny is smart to consider surgery when needed to keep hips, knees, and eyes functioning at a high level, without pain or dysfunction. I know whereof I speak. I'm here writing, sitting on two titanium hips and looking at the laptop screen through decataracted eyes that also had a nip and tuck at the same time to correct nearsightedness.

Eyes of a hawk. Who knew it could happen at this time of life? And who knew older women would turn out to be so darned improvable?

Finally, don't let fear keep you from correcting what might send you far too early to a rocking chair. Hot Granny, it's you who needs to rock—not the chair.

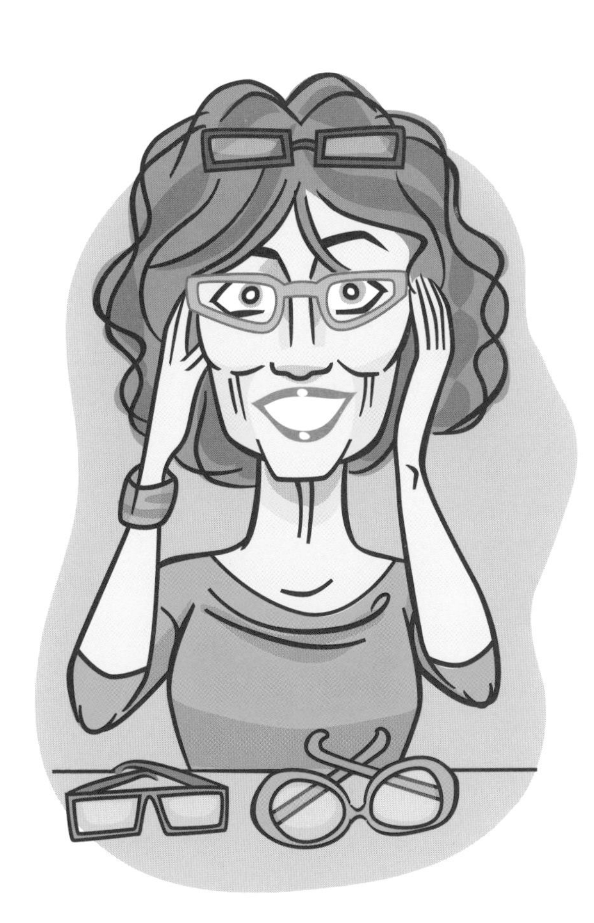

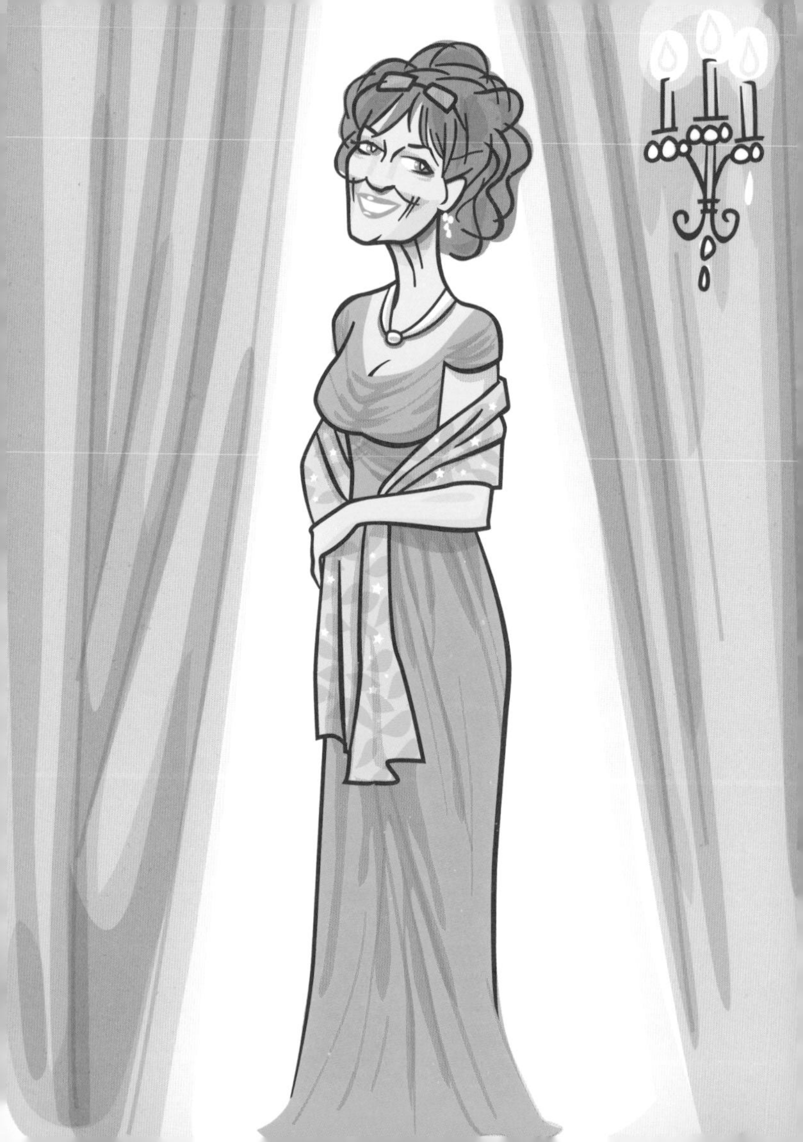

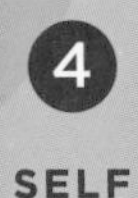

SELF

Looking and Feeling Like a Hot Granny

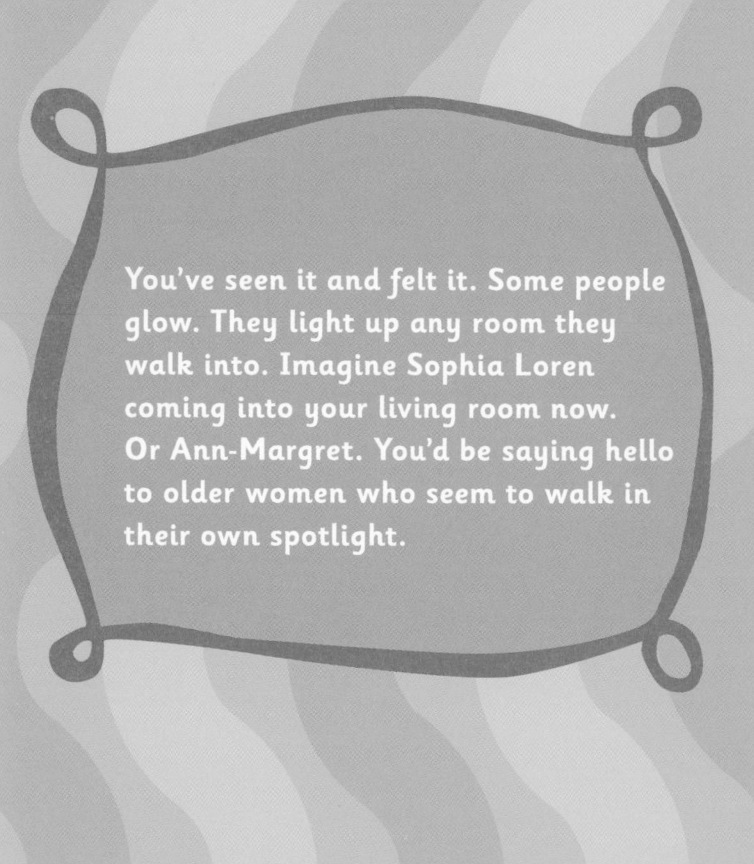
You've seen it and felt it. Some people glow. They light up any room they walk into. Imagine Sophia Loren coming into your living room now. Or Ann-Margret. You'd be saying hello to older women who seem to walk in their own spotlight.

The rest of us can generate our own starshine, the radiance that powers personal attraction. Sure, it's not world-class star power—few can put out that many watts. What we mortals can generate is more like the down-home charm that comes from respecting yourself enough to take care of the wonderful older woman that is you.

It's not frivolous to care how you look. You are beautifying the nation, cheering up your family, and keeping your own spirits high. Anyhow, the world expects older people to let themselves go—it's part of the negative stereotype—so surprise them.

What Makes a Woman Look and Feel Like a Hot Granny?

To look and feel like a Hot Granny, pay attention to these issues:

- **DEEP COMFORT**—BECAUSE IRRITATIONS CAN TAKE THE SHINE OFF HOT GRANNY.
- **GOOD SLEEP**—BECAUSE INSOMNIA CAN RUIN HOT GRANNY'S DAY.
- **GOOD LOOKS**—BECAUSE IT'S TIME TO BRING OUT THE VERY BEST OF HOT GRANNY.

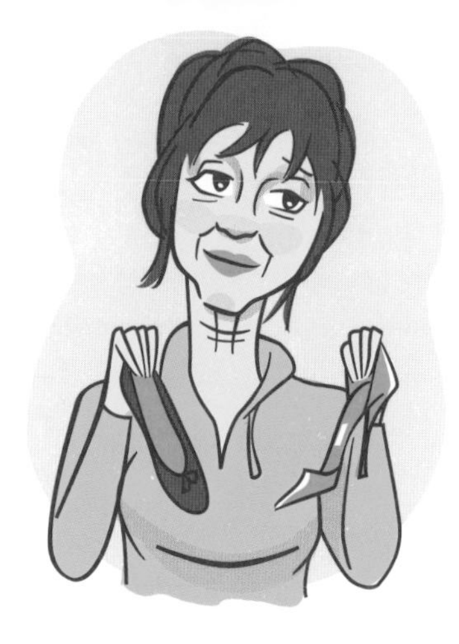

Deep Comfort

Start with simple basics, the physical underpinnings of comfort. The fact is, a Hot Granny won't be happy if her shoes are a size too small, if her bra cuts, or if her panties ride up. So here's how to keep irritation creep in check, leaving your Hot Granny self comfortable. Let's start at the bottom:

Shoes. Shoe sizes change over time. Feet flatten and widen. The *B* word—rhymes with *onion*—can widen the front of the foot. So have your tootsies remeasured, Cinderella, and stay away from glass slippers. Think flats or low heels. If you think flats and style don't go together, remember ballerinas. If they aren't stylish, who is?

Now, are you on your feet all day down at the salt mine? Then look for some of the popular European imports that the granola set found long ago—clogs and step-ins, shoes actually designed for comfort. Note that many comfort shoes now have style-shine and color-pizzazz. Think Hot Granny Red.

Some of us lose some of the padding on the bottom of our feet as we grow older. Padded socks come to the rescue here. You will find them near the sports shoes. They can put the spring back in your walk. Highly recommended.

Bras. Remember those training bras? 32 AA? Didn't need them, but wanted them. Well, you got trained and now may be a 42 D—boobs at last. But what about your bra ambitions today? Ha! Now you don't want them, but need them. Something has to keep the sisters in line.

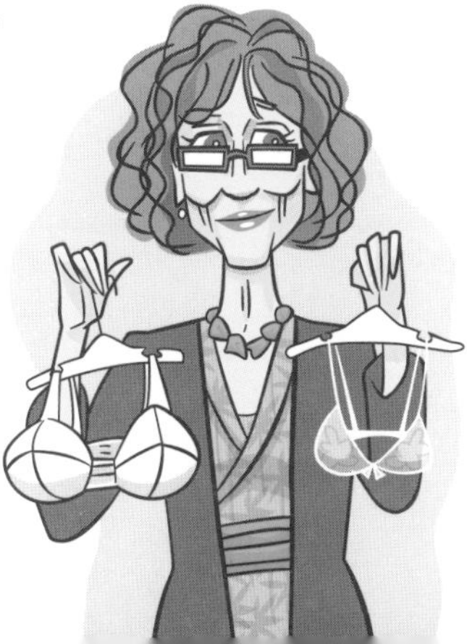

Many of us walk around in ill-fitting brassieres, constantly hiking straps up or yanking bands down. Why? Because we were a 34 B years ago but have morphed into a different size.

So get re-measured, or, if it just seems too weird to be alone in the dressing room with the lady and her measuring tape, get in there yourself with a range of bras. Try them on. Try color. Try lace. Try black and sexy. But, first and foremost, look for comfort. No more red lines around your chest or on your shoulders.

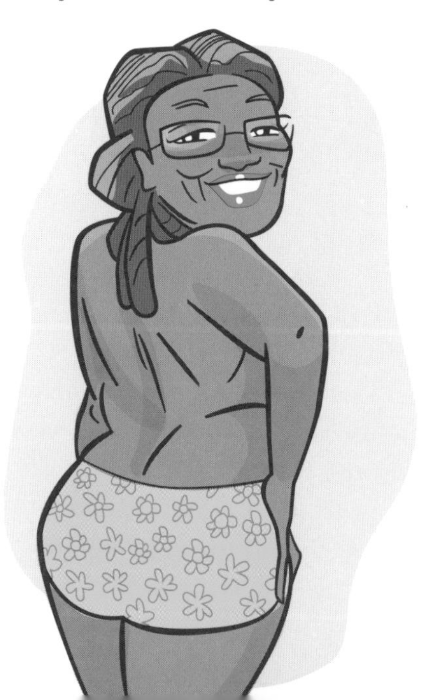

Panties. There is no universal law of nature that says older women must wear white cotton granny panties. Cotton is good because it keeps private parts healthy, but when it comes to style, go for color and florals. In this day and age, it's not hard to find styles that are both sexy and comfortable. Think how you will surprise the emergency-room staff after that accident your mom always warned you about.

And if you leak a little when you laugh, don't stop laughing. Just pick up a box of panty liners. If you leak a lot, see a doc. Leaks can be improved. Last, if your bumbershay has expanded, so has your panty size. Make sure it's the right size and comfortable for you.

What else will make you look and feel like a Hot Granny?

Good Sleep

Insomnia can ruin granny's day—and her night. Here's what to do if you can't sleep.

Check your mattress: Is it lumpy? Dead? If yes, go to a store and lie down on every mattress you can find. Do it. If you are single, do a solo act. If you're married, bring your mate. Either way, wear slacks and kick-off shoes. Get a feel for each kind of mattress—memory foam, sleep number, and pillow top. Sleep-numbered mattresses allow a couple to choose individual firmness levels.

Add a killer mattress pad: Mattress pads have gone upscale. Now there are thick quilted numbers, sometimes stuffed with down. Don't knock lying on a goose's coat until you try it. Heavenly.

Look to your sheets: You'll think you are turning into a princess-and-a-pea kind of gal when you learn to tell the difference between a high-thread-count sheet and the kind of sheets Mom used to buy. It's the difference between silk and sackcloth. Very soothing.

Play your tunes: Research confirms it—music helps you sleep. Slow music can even slow your breathing and respiration. But only you know exactly what kind of music will work.

To float away on your music and not wake up your mate, try an MP3 player with earphones. You can put all your CDs on one player, which is why people worship their iPods—all your beloved music in one pocket. These music players are highly recommended for Hot Granny, not just for insomnia but also for enriching life with your favorite music always at your fingertips. Such music players can be put into recharging holders that are also speakers; then the whole house can hear the music they were playing the year you met *him*.

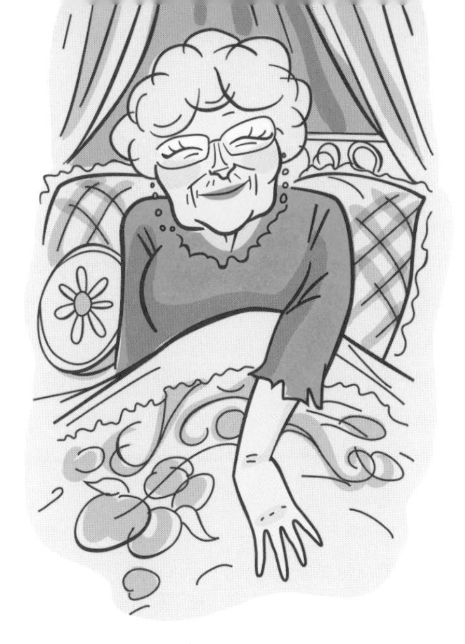

Outside exercise promotes sleep, so get out: It worked when you were a kid—didn't you sleep well?—and it can work now. Besides, a walk in the sunshine elevates mood and relieves depression. It is my belief that the human species now lives inside so much, it is giving itself seasonal affective disorder (SAD) all year 'round. To protect your skin, you can walk in the early morning or late in the day, when the sun is mild.

Investigate teas and potions: Check out the many kinds of relaxing, tension-taming teas. Experiment and see what works for you: chamomile, linden, valerian, gin?

Use your common sense: You'll hear some stupid "rules" about sleeping, such as that you are never to use your bedroom for anything except sleeping. But most women use their bedrooms for TV, manicures, arguments, daydreaming, exercise, wardrobe coordination, headaches, sex, phoning friends, entertaining, eating, reading books like this, and, yes, sleeping.

Now, what else can put a glow on a Hot Granny? Well, spend a minute in our department of good looks.

Good Looks

Looking good as an older woman doesn't mean you have to wear fashion reruns like miniskirts and go-go boots. Figure out what contemporary looks suit you, and stock your closet only with those pieces.

Dressing. It takes ten minutes a day to go from a lukewarm granny in her old bathrobe to someone who looks and feels like a Hot Granny. In the morning, instead of throwing on the clothes you wore yesterday, really think about what you're going to wear today. Then put on those well-chosen clothes.

Oh, I can hear you now: "I don't have anything to wear." What people may mean by this lament is that they don't have anything they *love* to wear. So, get rid of what you don't love, and find something you do.

Color. If you didn't do it in the 1980s, find your colors—the ones that bring out your eyes, complexion, and hair. Everybody has colors that they "own." Everybody. And if you did wear your colors in the 1980s, when they were fashionable, your colors may have changed.

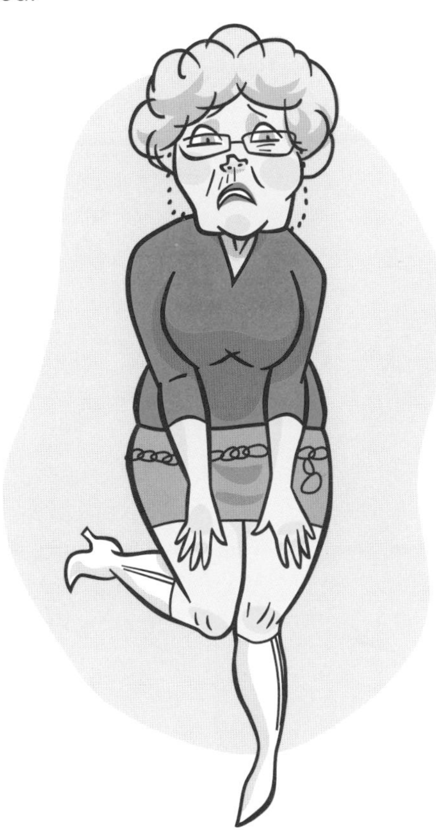

Your hair color may not be the same now, and your skin may have morphed into a lighter shade of pale. So, go to a store and hold up variously colored clothes in front of you as you look in a mirror. You don't have to try these on; you are looking for color only. Some colors will light you up. Others will dull you down or do nothing for you. See what makes you glow. Try colors you've never tried before, and then buy clothes in those colors. Don't forget deep purple, raspberry, red, and pink. Women with gray hair may be wise to move beyond their beige stage.

Style. Avoid granny style—think of Ruth Buzzi playing Gladys on *Laugh-In* and avoid your own Buzzification. No baggy cardigans, sagging hose, sculpted hard hair, or weird little purses. Pick a style that suits you, and stick to it. And pick a clothes mentor.

Maybe Julie Andrews or Diane Sawyer, with their simple but stylish charm? Or are you Sally Field—perky? How about Susan Sarandon, simple but sexy? Just don't dress like the stereotype of yesterday's granny, or that's how you'll be treated—someone who should stay home and soak her bunions in vinegar water.

Buy the good classic pieces rather than bargain-bin junk that doesn't fit, doesn't feel good, and that you don't love. And remember what good accessories can do for your clothes and your spirits.

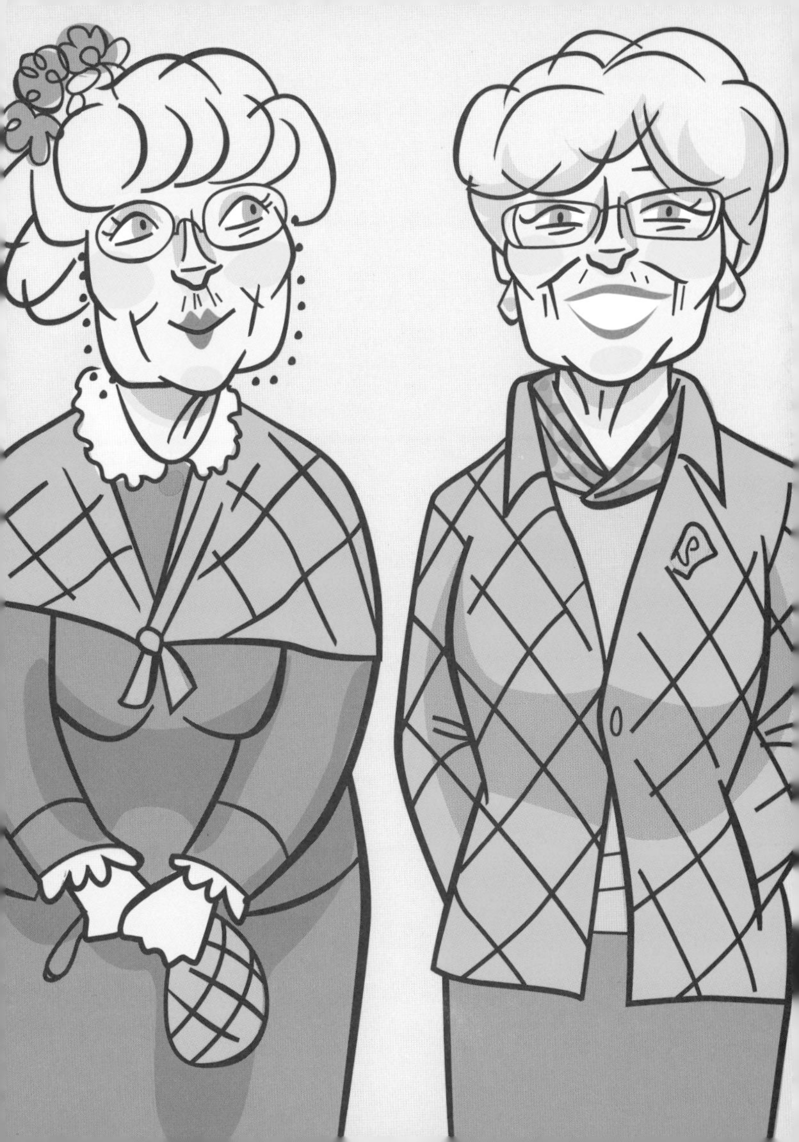

Hair. Let us turn now to Major Hair Sins, and the greatest of them is dry, lusterless hair. Please don't give up on shiny hair just because you are a grandmother. Give your hair conditional love—lots of conditioner. And don't rinse your hair blue or go for uptight curls. Get a good haircutter and a good haircut that fits your face and style. Color your hair if you want, but consider the easy glories of silver hair. If you do color, don't go for very dark hair if you are Caucasian. It looks artificial next to pale skin. Some women go blonder and slowly morph into white hair.

Cosmetics. Makeup has changed. Get a free cosmetic-counter makeover and see which products light up your face. Buy only those products. Don't be pushed into buying more. Younger females in your family can be helpful in steering you toward what looks great.

Argue if you want, but makeup can make a huge difference in your appeal as a Hot Granny. And yes, I know all about the appeal of the freshly washed face with nothing on it. That was when we were fifteen.

Finally, use lots of light and a magnifying mirror. And don't stop the foundation at the bottom of your face. You have a neck. Conceal it.

Skin. Moisturize your hide twice a day. If you want to get the wrinkles out with peels and injections, do it, but can you think of other ways to spend that time and money? One of the dangers of peels, injections, and plastic surgery is that the industry may convince you that you are worthless without its products or services—that every wrinkle is a blot upon the soul.

Some of the women on TV, with their featureless, drawn-back faces, look like aliens from outer space to me, but the choice is up to you. You can let your face settle nicely where it wants or take it a few steps back. I'm a settler. Easy, inexpensive, no side effects.

There is one easy fix: A dermatologist can remove those brown age spots from your face in a few minutes. Yes, it stings, and yes, it's worth it. Don't go to just any dermatologist in the phone book. Get a referral from a satisfied client.

Grooming. Some of us older women have a shelf on our chests. It's the shelf of the ample mammaries. You can bet that shelf will be hit by drops of pasta sauce on their way to the floor. So, you gotta check your front shelf. I know, I know—men have been doing that for you all your life, but now you have to patrol for food spots. Try not to spill in the first place. Attend to any spots so that you won't walk around looking demented—Ms. Spots on Her Shirt. Poor thing.

And take care of those stray hairs that may be sprouting from surprising places—eyebrows, chin,

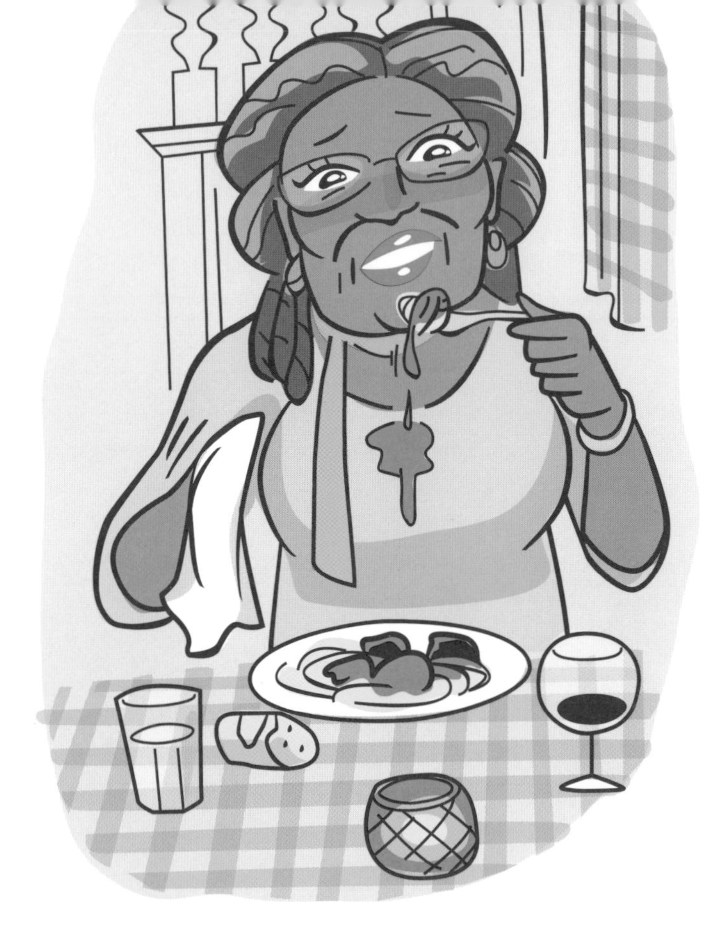

nose, ears. Who knew? Some women snip or shave, others bleach, and still others wax, depending on the area. But don't have a fit over the new little hairs on your chinny chin chin. Just take care of them.

Body language. Shoulders back and light on your feet. Hot Granny doesn't slump her way across life's stage. Remember that Carly Simon line: "You walked into the party like you were walking onto a yacht." If that's vanity—to walk proud—I'll have another helping, please.

How to Keep the Glow

Take all the above, and repeat.

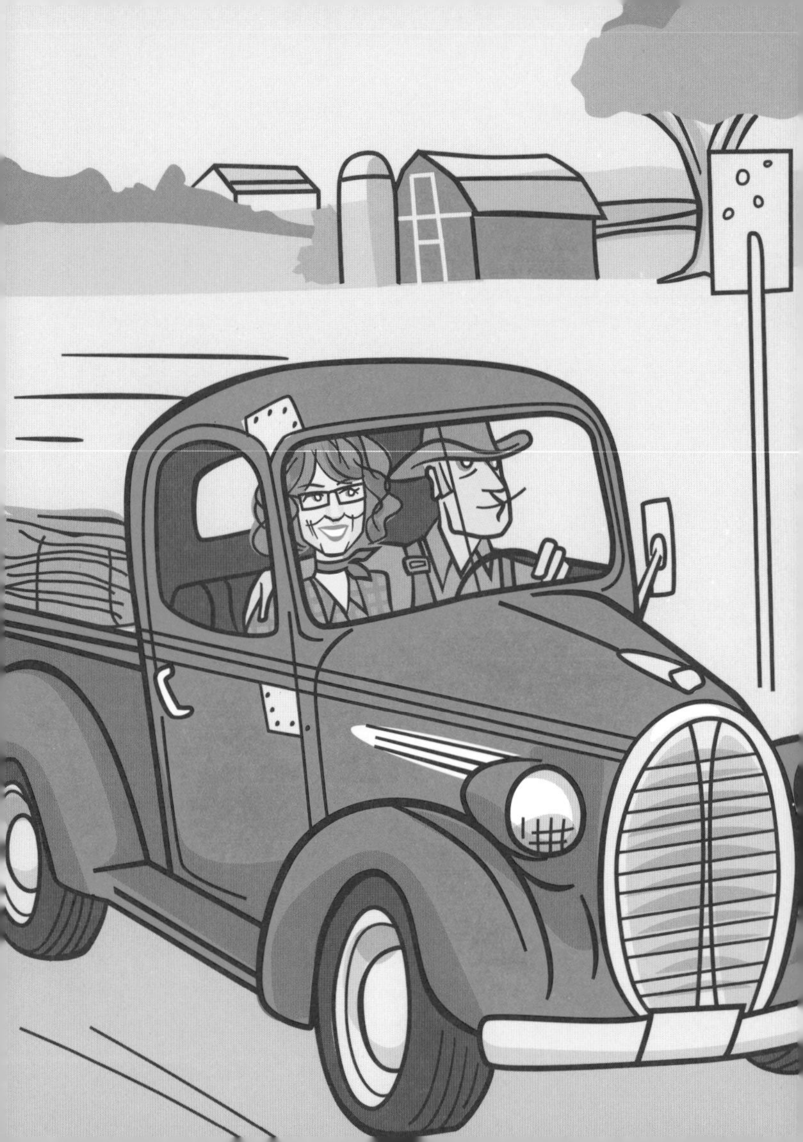

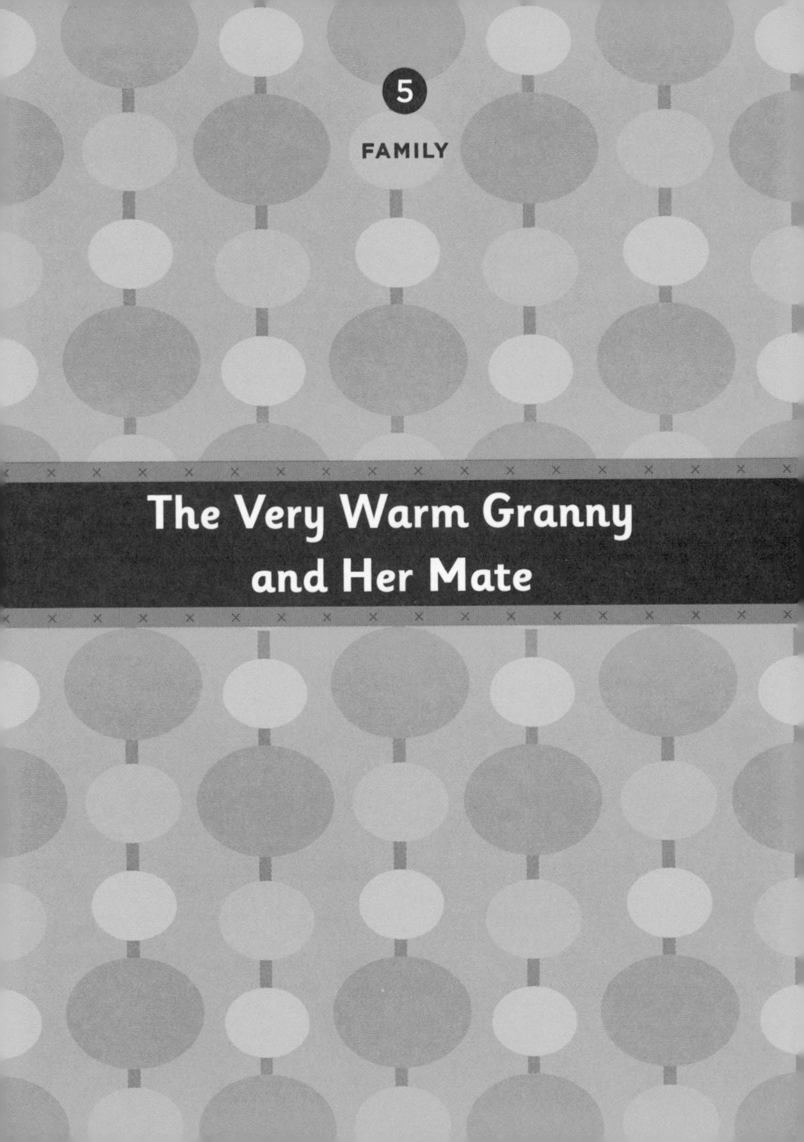
5
FAMILY
The Very Warm Granny
and Her Mate

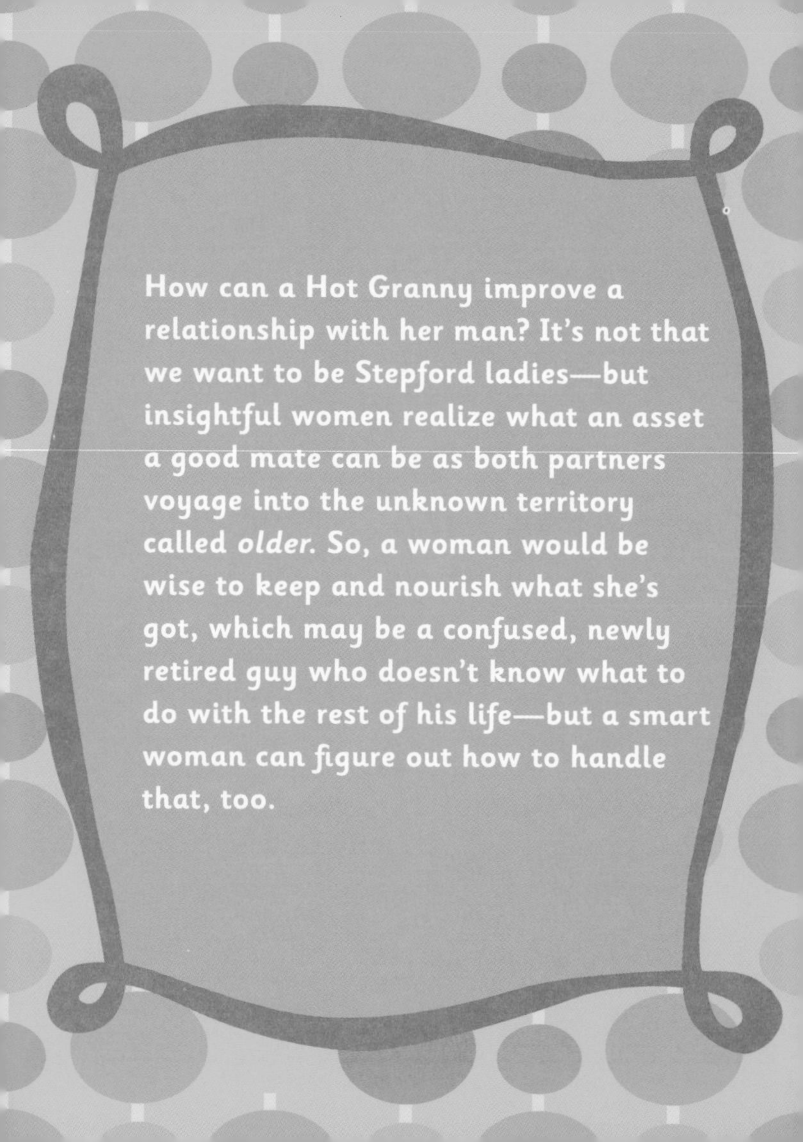

How can a Hot Granny improve a relationship with her man? It's not that we want to be Stepford ladies—but insightful women realize what an asset a good mate can be as both partners voyage into the unknown territory called *older*. So, a woman would be wise to keep and nourish what she's got, which may be a confused, newly retired guy who doesn't know what to do with the rest of his life—but a smart woman can figure out how to handle that, too.

Hot Granny's Rules for Loving a Guy with Gray Hair

Offer praise and acknowledgment—especially if the mate in question is newly retired. He now has no colleagues to tell him he's doing well. As one retired man notes: "I lost my audience." So, guess who's left to clap when the applause of the workplace has been taken away? You. Also lost is a large chunk of his identity. Until retirement, he was an engineer or a salesman or a pharmacist, and now he is not. Yes, he is your husband, but that identity has been enough for only one person in the world—Queen Elizabeth's man. Until your mate gets his teeth into interesting retirement activities, you are his main source of recognition. So think of yourself as a one-woman Nobel committee. Give prizes.

Avoid criticism—for all the reasons above. And if you have bones to pick, do it privately. Do it delicately, rarely, and with good humor. Consider the insult sandwich as a way of delivering criticism. Insult sandwich? That would be a compliment followed by a layer of criticism and finished with a top layer of compliment. Compliment, criticism, compliment—you can do that.

Leave him alone sometimes. A Hot Granny experienced in love knows what men really want besides hot sex and cold martinis. Men want to be left alone. They want time to themselves to do anything they want, and that includes doing nothing. They want time to watch football, baseball, and westerns without having to bargain, beg, or feel they are being "allowed" to watch.

Communicate with consideration. Don't hog the phone, or, if you collide over phone calls, get two lines.

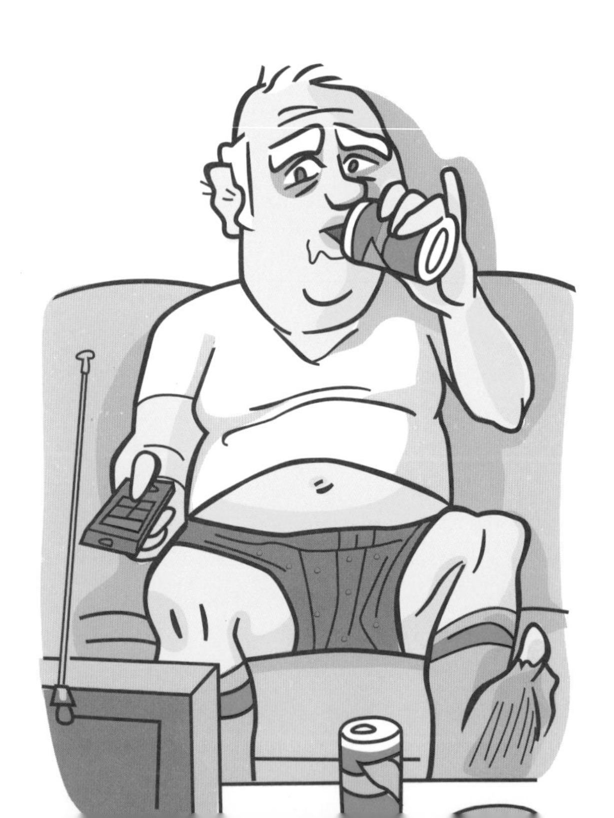

And don't talk to him from the other room. It drives him crazy because he can't hear. Heck, now he may not even be able to hear when you are in the same room, and he may resist hearing aids. Refusing to get hearing aids is a source of many an argument. Be patient. He can't cover them with hair the way you can.

What's also crazy-making is him talking on the phone while you're in the background telling him what to say. Getting a phone with a speaker function solves this problem. You can then have a three-way simultaneous conversation with anyone.

Look presentable—even if the tired part of you says nobody cares. He does, and actually, you do, too. No Hot Granny wants to look or feel like a bag lady. See chapter 4, "Looking and Feeling Like a Hot Granny."

Be a buddy, ready and willing to get up, go, and enjoy things together—travel, theater, music, whatever. The world is waiting for you both, and sad is the older man who at last has the time to hit the road but no willing mate to go with him. Not that you have to do everything together, but some common things are essential if you want to stay in touch with each other's joys and hiking blisters.

Be affectionate—in and out of bed. Read on for the sex part.

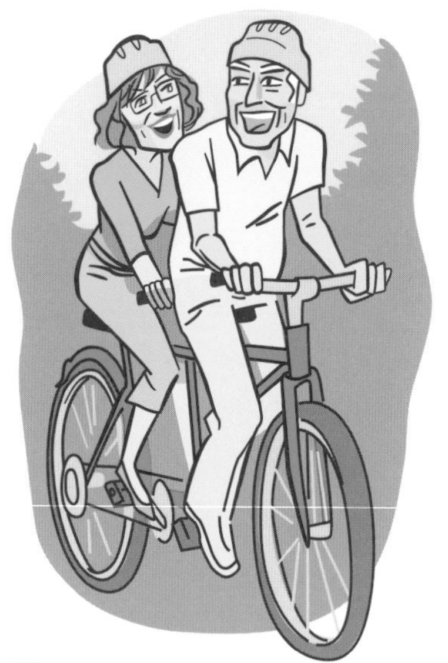

The Sex Part

Turn fifty, lose it—that's the stereotype. The truth is, some people lose it at thirty—never liked sex, never will—and some people keep the fire burning until they go out the door, toes up. As long as there's life, there can be sex. And that's the carnal aspiration of a Hot Granny: to keep the fires going.

Why do people have trouble believing that older people like sex? Maybe because they can't imagine their parents in bed—too threatening—and so they generalize this sexless image and impose it on all older people.

But common sense should tell anyone that if a man still has a penis and a woman still has a clitoris, then they have all they need for continued pleasure. You don't need a prescription to use your parts or a license to take them out for a spin. The pleasure parts of the body are free, available 24/7, and with you all your life.

Lovemaking in later life can be more satisfying than in the days of your shy youth. By now you know what you like and may be more willing to ask for it. Maybe you don't worry so much now about cellulite. And maybe he can't see much without his glasses. Freedom from judgment at last.

Barriers to Good Sex and How to Break Through

Just as there were barriers to sex when you were young (parents and unwanted pregnancy) and just as there were barriers to sex in midlife (kids and fatigue), so there are barriers in later life. Yes, you now have the privacy—no kids walking in. But there are glitches to consider. Here are some common problems of the older couple and what you can do about them.

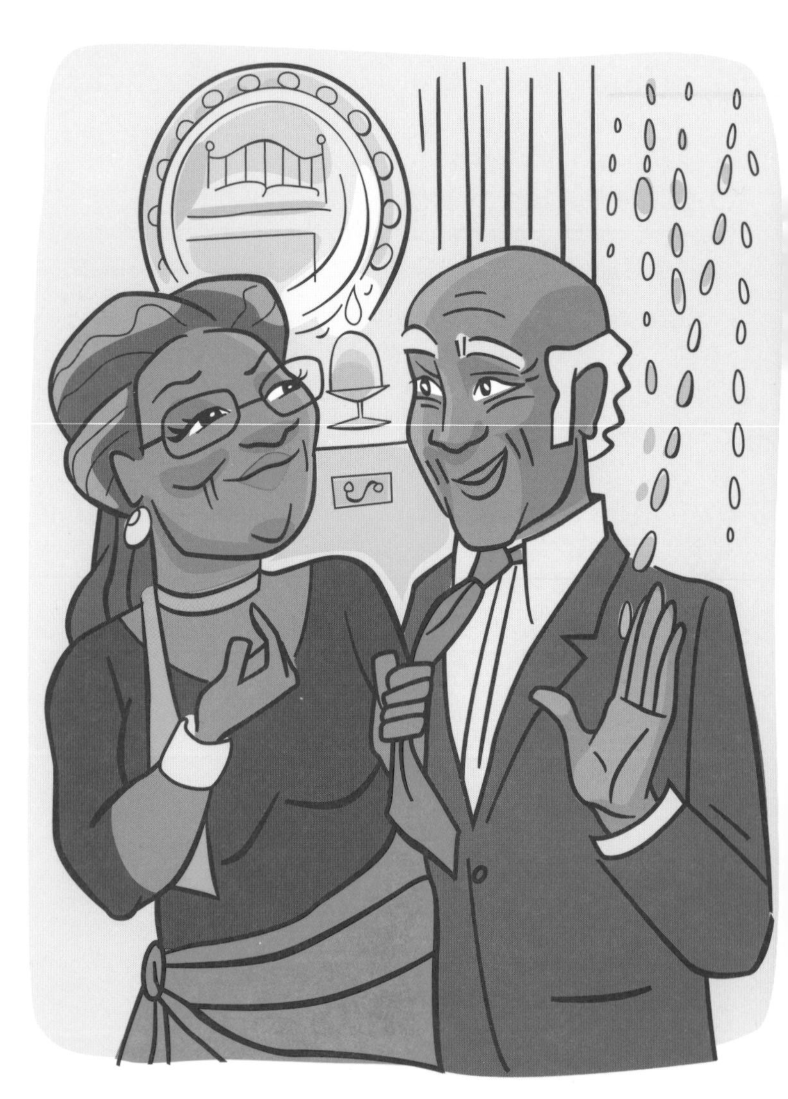

CHANGES IN SEXUAL EQUIPMENT

Expect change. Your man's private parts may be slower to spring into action. This is not your fault. If an older man has circulatory problems, those problems can extend to his extender. The blood won't flow freely into the penis, and that blood flow is, after all, what powers the Erector set. Also, medications can change blood flow. Remember, blood-pressure meds lower the pressure in the *whole* body. So, medications can change behavior.

As for erection time and quality, my read is that these changes upset men far more than women, especially any change in firmness. It's why men buy drugs for erectile dysfunction (ED). Some men have little dysfunction but a great desire to replicate the old days in bed. Men may think they have the fountain of youth in a pill, and to some extent they are right. But all drugs have side effects.

Keep an eye on the pharmaceutical news, and read the inserts that are part of the drug package. Note that Viagra has been associated with permanent loss of vision. Serious stuff. So these pills are not toys. Incidentally, Medicare now covers pills for ED.

Your tax dollars at work.

THE CHALLENGES OF LATER-LIFE LOVE

Later-life love offers rewards, but the challenges are there, too. For instance, intercourse may be a little more difficult for older adults, not like sliding into home plate anymore. Either or both partners may be having trouble in the parts department. As noted, he may have trouble getting or maintaining his erection. Her vagina may be too dry to comfortably receive it. Either (or both) may have physical issues that interfere—osteoporosis, arthritis, obesity, diabetes, post-surgical vulnerabilities, and heart concerns. But if there are two wills, there's a way. Probably several ways.

People can get very inventive when getting around physical limitations. If you run out of ideas, look at one of those books where humans do pretzel thingies in bed. But don't rip a muscle, pop a vertebra, or do anything that hurts either one of you.

Now, if a Hot Granny needs help with lubrication, she can find it in the drugstore section that carries the intimate stuff like condoms. And if she wants a home-made lube solution, she doesn't have to look further than her own kitchen for the simple answer of cooking oil. (Add a touch of vanilla extract to canola oil, and beg for a body massage while you're at it.)

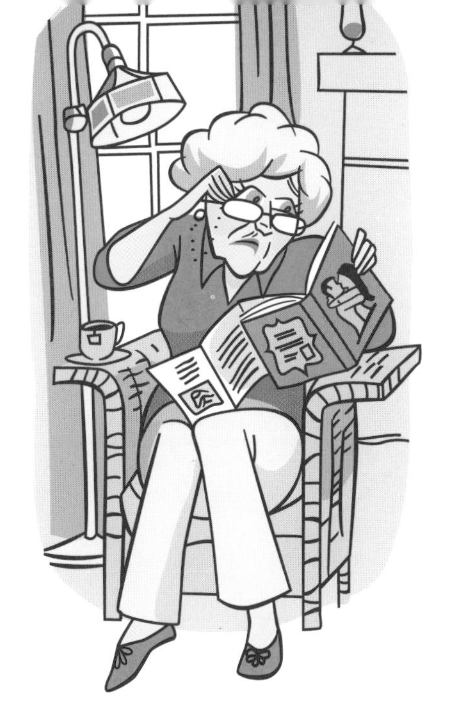

LIBIDO LOSS

Granny and her honey may need a few sex helpers to kick off their libidos. Do not be afraid to go bravely into the world of video to giggle at the bad movie-making, the phony female orgasms, and the impossibly large-membered men who sign on for this kind of video work. Such fare is probably available on your home TV. If it turns you off, remember: You are the ruler of the remote.

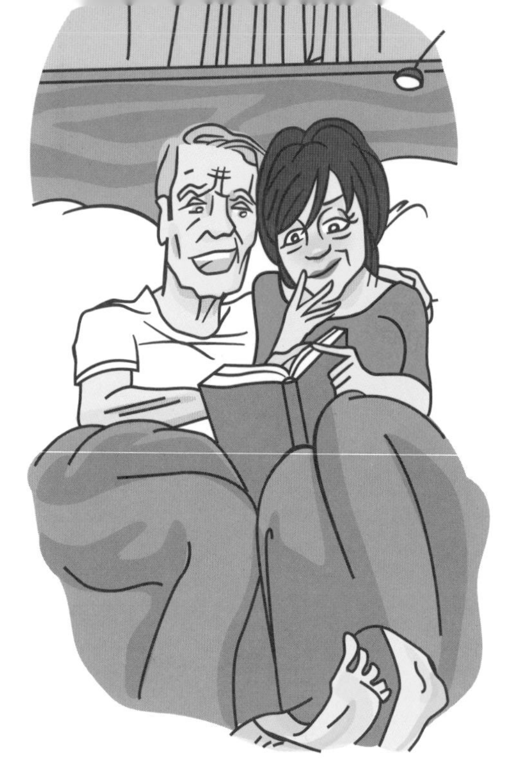

Other ways to get in the mood: giving and getting a body massage, reading erotica together, planning romantic nights or weekends away, surprising him with a gift of sexy shorts, or using vibrators or other sex toys. If you want inspiration, you'll find it at www.goodvibes.com, where they teach how to "tickle his pickle" and much, much more. And don't miss www.a-womans-touch.com.

Don't forget that sex can be a pleasant do-it-yourself proposition. Consider masturbation as a way of exercising your orgasmic abilities. Orgasms are not rationed, and the more you have, the more you may want to have.

The Attitude-Gratitude Part

Every relationship has its stresses—the down days, the sulks and silences. That's natural enough when the relationship is cross-gender, which it usually is—male and female, Mars and Venus, different worlds trying to make one world together. To a woman who values intimacy and companionship, the effort is worth the result. If any reader wants to remind herself how lucky she is that her man still inhabits the earth, she should listen to her widowed friends.

Yes, some widows make great adjustments, run with a pack of interesting female friends, and even find a new mate, but there are widows who are forlorn, who feel shut out of the couples' world. I was a divorced woman for many years, and I well remember those Sunday mornings when it seemed every satisfied couple in the world was out for brunch. And then there was me—eggs Benedict for one.

Notice how much social life is couples-oriented—dances, parties, bridge, travel. A Noah's-ark social life can be hard on the single woman who doesn't have some survival strategies in her playbook. (Chapter 2, "Granny Single, Granny Hot," tells the divorced and widowed how to navigate the social waters alone.)

My point is that every older woman who has a living, breathing, high-quality mate should give thanks to the domestic gods that he continues to exist. Statistically, he will graduate from the planet before she does. Every single day counts. Make that every hour.

So, for the happily mated Hot Granny, these are the good old days. And the even better news is that she and her mate have a chance to live another lifetime. A hundred years ago, the average age at death was in the late forties. Now people live into their eighties. Such marvelous longevity is unprecedented in human history. Not to take advantage of this demographic miracle is a waste. Enjoy the gift of time. These extra years allow us the space to catch life's second wind.

As you know from this book's introduction, I host a radio show for older adults. I call the show *Second Wind* because that's what today's older adults can enjoy as they move from middle age to life beyond. And when it comes to relationships, life's second wind is a breath of fresh air that can revive a veteran marriage or even foster a new relationship. As my husband and I said at our recent wedding, "At our age, 'until death do us part' is doable."

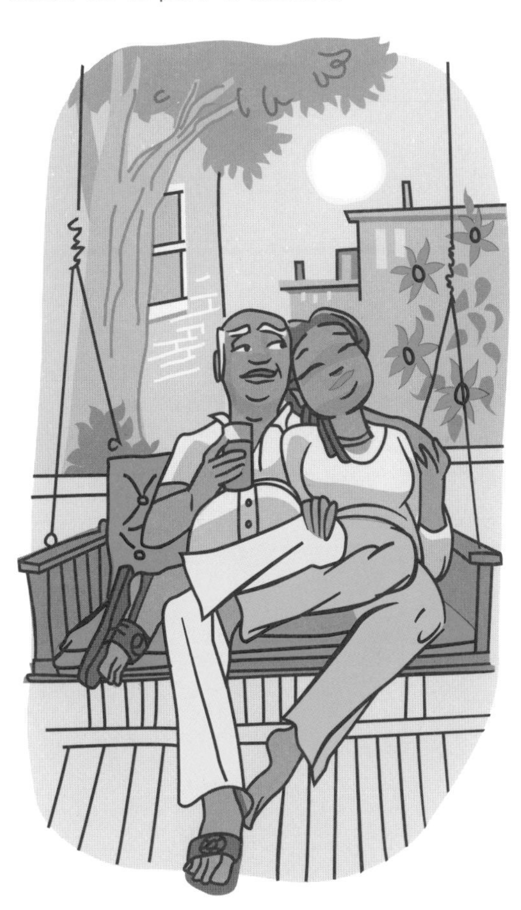

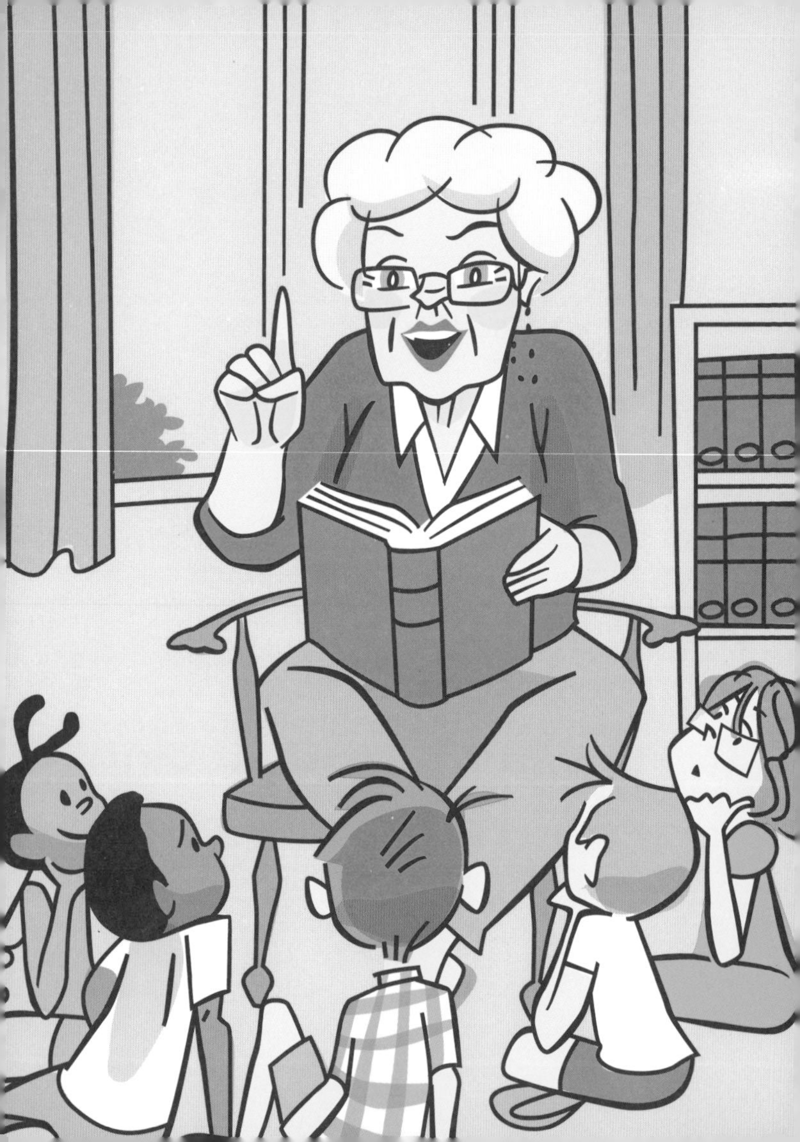

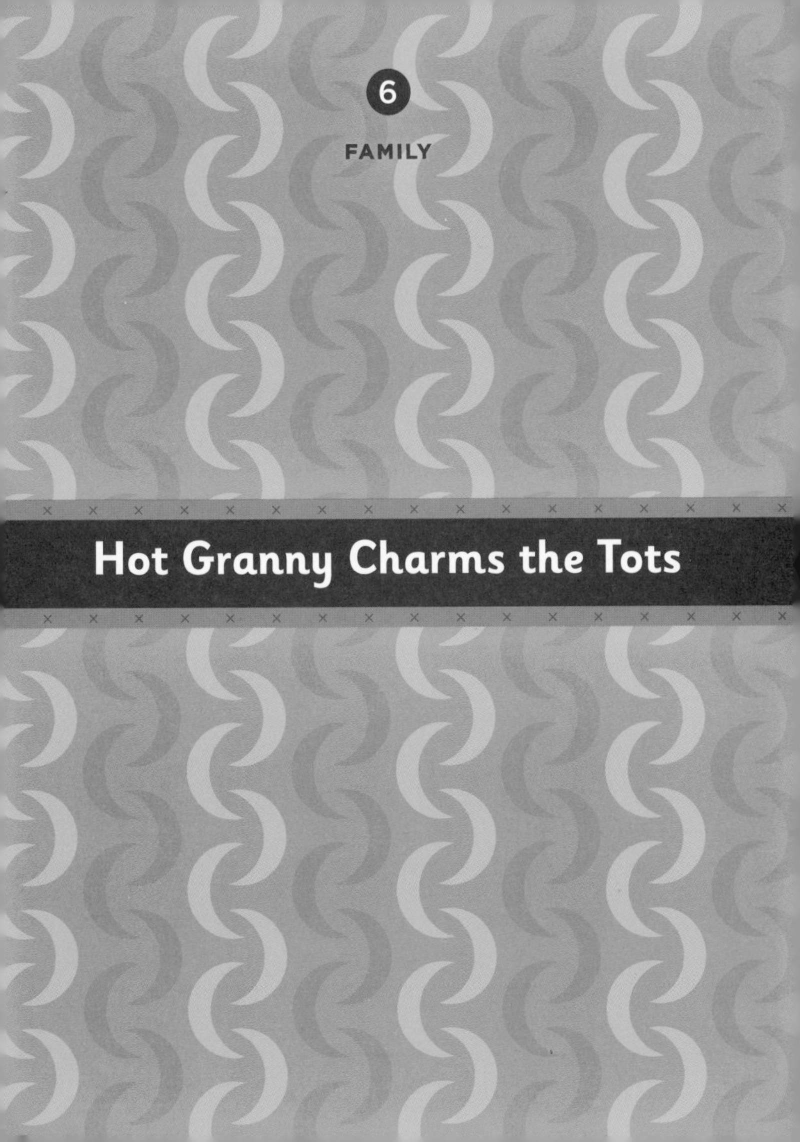

6

FAMILY

Hot Granny Charms the Tots

A Hot Granny cares about the youngest generation. And she doesn't need to have a blood-relative grandchild to be a nurturing Hot Granny. Some older women do not have children or never married. Others have sons and daughters who have no kids. So, they are technically not grandmothers. Except in my book. I say any older woman who helps the youngest generation turn out right is a very Hot Granny indeed.

And don't most of us—whatever our life circumstance—feel some obligation as senior members of the species to spend a little time and effort mentoring young humans into personhood?

That is easier said than done, I know. Families scatter coast-to-coast. Airplane travel to see grandchildren can be stressful and expensive. Sometimes the parent does not encourage contact, which makes it hard to be close to the younger generation. Plus, the kids and their parents are overscheduled, which leaves little time for grandparent visits. And phone calls, when they do come, can seem awkward. "Here, say something to Granny"—when the grandson would rather play with his Game Boy or other tech toy.

And you should know this: No matter what you do for or with your grandchildren, you probably will never be as interesting to them as an iPod. But once you know where you stand in the hierarchy of Things That Interest Kids, you won't have the expectation that you are their first priority. This is normal kid thinking, and just because we may rate a little lower than mac and cheese on the priority scale right now—well, that's no reason to give up on the young ones.

Remember what your priorities used to be? Kicking the can and ice-skating with other kids were my top priorities for years. And just because we are not the center of a grandchild's world doesn't mean we can't connect and have fun with him or her—maybe providing a little life instruction along the way.

What If Hot Granny Has No Grandkids?

As long as the world has children, any older woman will have small people to nurture. Yes, they may not be lab-certified blood grandchildren, but that doesn't lessen the experience. In fact, it makes the experience more remarkable. You become a grandmother by choice, not chance. You don't have to make those cookies or take them to Disneyland. You are a free-will Hot Granny.

If you want to find small people to help along in life, grandnieces and grandnephews may be a good place to start. Kids in the neighborhood are another option. Some people work with Big Brothers Big Sisters and set up a more formal system of mentoring. Others volunteer teaching or coaching. Whatever works.

The Reluctant Grandmother

Some women have a little nagging doubt about their status as grandmothers. Aren't I too young to be a grandmother? Or too involved in a career to do a good job at it? And aren't I way beyond the lace-tatting, pie-baking, gray-haired granny in the ads?

These are some of the questions, and each of us answers in her own way. One answer is to realize that few believe the granny stereotypes anymore. They are out-of-date and increasingly out-of-mind. Another solution is to realize that grannyhood is not motherhood. One of the pleasures of this time of life is that the painful choices between career and family are rare. There's time and space for both now, and you can embrace grandmotherhood without giving up who you are and what you like to do.

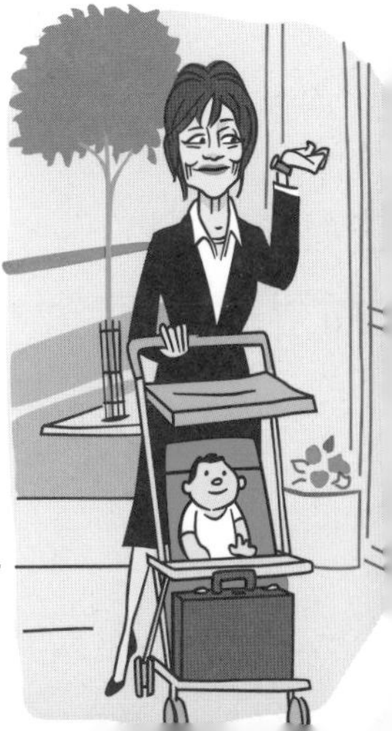

Still other women just don't like the sound of *Grandma*, and so they invent other names for themselves. This process can be fun and go way beyond *Nana* or *Granny*. So, select a name for yourself, and don't be surprised if "the other grandmother" takes your first choice. Don't get mad. Get another name.

Making Connections: One Hundred Hot Grannies Tell How

Shared pleasant experiences are one key to making a connection with grandkids. Traveling, sharing family celebrations, learning about their good deeds in school, watching them at their sports—all these things foster connection. Doing puzzles, playing cards and games, and looking at movies together are also winners—especially movies, for they are the shared vocabulary of the twenty-first century—stories on the screen that all ages can relate to and remember as something special.

But what movies? So many of them seem violent, stupid, and not worth the rental money or the time. Well, I asked a hundred Hot Grannies—an online group of college classmates—and they came up with some excellent ideas, which I now pass on to you.

The next time you want to set up a time of popcorn and shared fun (and not be bored silly), order one of these films:

The African Queen, An American in Paris, Bambi, Beauty and the Beast, Bend It Like Beckham, Carousel, Cinderella, Dances with Wolves, Eight Below, Finding Nemo, Hidalgo,

The King and I, Lassie Come Home, The Lion King, The Man from Snowy River, Meet Me in St. Louis, The Music Man, National Velvet, Oklahoma!, The Princess Diaries (1 and 2), **The Red Shoes, The Right Stuff, Seabiscuit, Shane, Singin' in the Rain, South Pacific,** any **Wallace and Gromit** title, **West Side Story,** or **The Whale Rider.**

As for games, you either like games or you hate them. If you hate them, don't play them. If you like them, try the following recommended games—more tested ideas from the hundred Hot Grannies:

Bingo, Boggle, Cadoo, Chutes and Ladders, Crazy Eights, Go Fish, Jenga, Monopoly, Old Maid, Parcheesi, Scrabble, Set, or **Sorry.** Some of these games can also be played online.

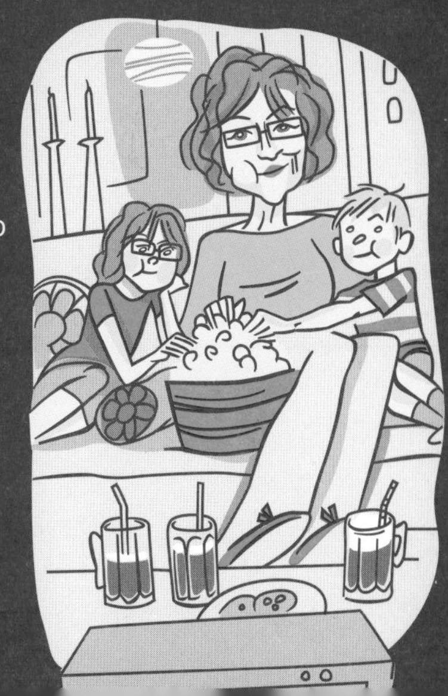

Bonus points for any Hot Granny: if you are hip to video gaming, your grandchild will be astonished. At least ask your grandkids for a demo of the current games. Advanced cybergrannies can even play video games with grandkids over the Internet.

When You Visit Your Grandchildren: The Rules

Visits can be fun, or visits can be a drag on one or both sides. Here are some things to ponder as you pack your suitcase to visit the kids at their home.

- **THIS IS NOT YOUR HOUSE, AND THESE ARE NOT YOUR RULES.** GO BY THE RULES YOUR CHILDREN HAVE ESTABLISHED FOR THEIR HOUSEHOLDS. IF YOU QUESTION THESE RULES, KEEP YOUR OPINION TO YOURSELF. GO WITH THE FLOW. YOU MIGHT LEARN SOMETHING.

- **BRING A LITTLE PRESENT** FOR EACH KID AND ONE FOR THE HOUSEHOLD.

- **TAKE THEM OUT FOR A MEAL OR TWO.** AND OFFER TO COOK A MEAL SO THE CHEF OF THE HOUSE WON'T HAVE TO. OR OFFER TO ORDER IN PIZZA.

- **DO NOT KEEP YOUR RECREATIONAL LIQUIDS ON THE REFRIGERATOR DOOR.** THIS INCLUDES GIN FOR YOUR NIGHTLY MARTINI. SERIOUSLY, LITTLE KIDS CAN THINK GROWN-UP TREATS ARE DRINKS FOR THEM. KEEP ALCOHOL OUT OF THEIR ORBIT.

- **IF YOU TAKE MEDICATIONS,** MAKE SURE NO LITTLE ONE CAN GET INTO YOUR SUITCASE OR PURSE.

- **OFFER TO BABYSIT** SO THE PARENTS CAN HAVE A DATE NIGHT.

- **ENTERTAIN YOURSELF** SO YOU WON'T BE AN ENERGY SINK. BRING BOOKS, WRITE IN A JOURNAL, LISTEN TO MUSIC, TAKE WALKS, OR TAKE THE KIDS SOMEWHERE.

- **IF YOU DRIVE THE KIDS ANYWHERE,** ALWAYS USE THE CAR SEATS AND SEAT BELTS. MANY OF US DROVE ACROSS THE COUNTRY WITH INFANTS IN OUR LAPS. NOT A GOOD IDEA THEN AND NOT A GOOD IDEA NOW.

- **THE ROMANS HAD IT RIGHT:** GUESTS AND FISH SMELL AFTER THREE DAYS. EVEN THE BEST FISH. EVEN THE BEST GUEST. SO, MOVE ON AND OUT, AND GO TORTURE THE NEXT SET OF FAMILY MEMBERS.

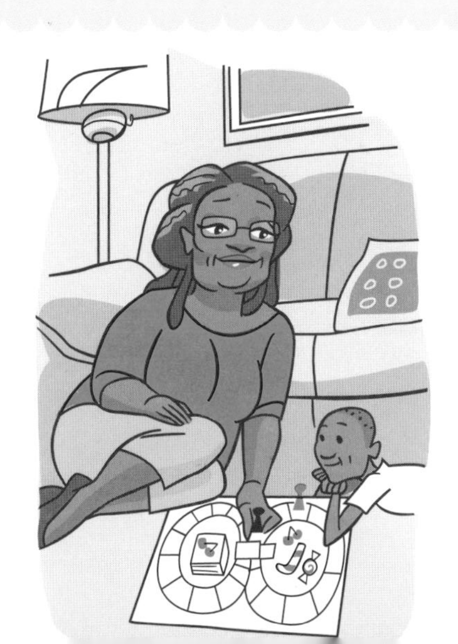

When They Visit You: The Rules

There are ways to make houseguests happy and the visit a success. Here are some ideas.

- **WELCOME THEM WITH A TREAT:** HOT CHOCOLATE, LUNCH, FLOWERS, A CHEERY HOUSE. DEAL WITH ANY STALE SMELLS. KIDS REMEMBER HOW THE HOUSES OF GRANDPARENTS SMELL.

- **FLUFF UP THE GUEST QUARTERS** AS BEST YOU CAN: CLEAN SHEETS AND TOWELS, LIGHTS BY THE BED, A PLACE TO PUT SUITCASES OR HANG CLOTHES.

- **IF YOU ARE SHORT ON BEDROOMS,** INFLATABLE BEDS ON THE FLOOR ARE HITS WITH KIDS. THAT AND A SLEEPING BAG ARE FINE. BUY AN INFLATABLE BED DESIGNED SO KIDS CAN'T ROLL OUT OF IT EASILY.

- **PULL-OUT COUCHES** ARE GREATLY IMPROVED BY A LAYER OF FOAM PADDING UNDER THE SHEETS.

- **IF A VISITING CHILD IS STILL LEAKING AT NIGHT,** PUT A SHOWER CURTAIN UNDER THE SHEET TO PROTECT THE MATTRESS. DIAPERS DO NOT ALWAYS FULLY CONTAIN THE LITTLE ONE'S NIGHT DEPOSITS.

- **FIND OUT IF ANYONE IS ALLERGIC** TO CERTAIN FOODS, TO ANIMALS, OR TO DOWN. ACT ACCORDINGLY. YOU DON'T HAVE TO GIVE THE CAT AWAY, BUT YOU DO HAVE TO VACUUM BEFORE AND KEEP

THE CAT CONFINED FOR THE DURATION OF THE VISIT. IF YOU LIKE YOUR CAT MORE THAN YOUR FAMILY, YOU HAVE ISSUES, DARLIN'.

- **PLAN ENTERTAINMENT.** GET SOME GOOD MOVIES AND GAMES. SEE THE LISTS ON PAGES 92–93.

- **ASK YOUR GRANDCHILDREN ABOUT THEIR LIVES.** ASK THEM TO SHOW YOU HOW THEIR TOYS WORK. GET A LEGO LECTURE, OR LEARN SOMETHING ABOUT A SONY PLAYSTATION. LOOK UP SOMETHING TOGETHER ON WWW.GOOGLE.COM: THEIR SCHOOL WEB SITE, WHERE THEY ARE GOING NEXT SUMMER, WHAT THEY WANT AS A HOLIDAY PRESENT.

- **IF JUST ONE GRANDCHILD IS GOING TO VISIT YOU,** FIND ANOTHER GRANDCHILD OR ANOTHER CHILD COMPANION. THOUGH WE HOT GRANNIES MAY BE DELIGHTFUL COMPANY, WE ARE NOT SO HOT AT PLAYING TAG, VIDEO GAMES, OR SNOWBOARDING. KIDS LIKE KIDS. THEY CAN GET LONESOME WITHOUT PEER COMPANIONSHIP. REMEMBER *ON GOLDEN POND.*

- **ONE OF THE BEST PRESENTS YOU CAN GIVE** YOUR OWN CHILDREN IS TO ACKNOWLEDGE THEIR SKILL AS PARENTS. SOME OF THEM ARE SUCH GOOD PARENTS, THEY SHOULD GET SPECIAL RECOGNITION. IT IS PROBABLY HARDER TO BRING UP KIDS TODAY THAN WHEN WE DID IT, SO SPEAK UP AND LET THEM KNOW THEY ARE DOING A GREAT JOB PRODUCING FIRST-RATE KIDS.

General Hot Granny Wisdom

Stay up-to-date. Learn something about computers and music players.

If you are staying away from computers or music players out of fear or unfamiliarity, you are missing a great way to connect with grandchildren. As my oldest granddaughter, Sydney, wrote to me:

"It would be nice if grandparents knew more about technology because it is such a major degree of separation between generations. It's difficult to explain the appeal of a video game to grandparents when they have no idea what it is or does for us. Knowledge of popular culture and technology really makes a grandparent seem up-to-date and more accessible."

So, Hot Granny, make yourself more accessible and learn some tech stuff. Knowing how to e-mail is becoming mainstream when it comes to grandparenting skills. Colleges and community centers offer many cybercourses. Computers are becoming cheaper all the time.

Keep this next rule in mind. It will help you get along with your children, who are, after all, the gatekeepers to your grandchildren:

Let everybody in the family live his or her own life.

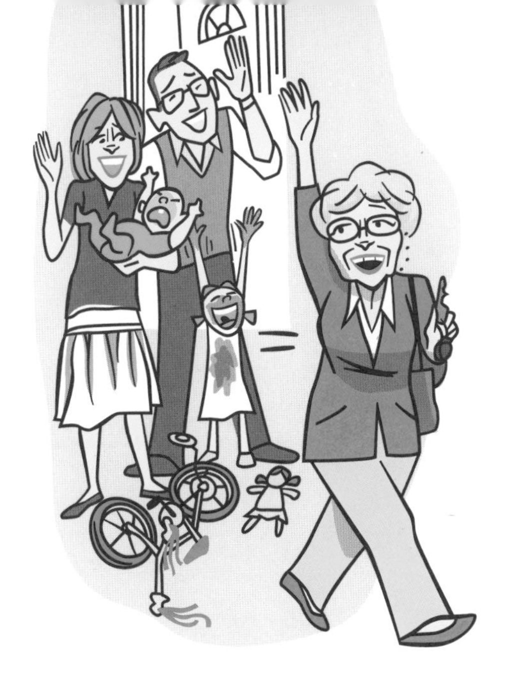

And others should extend this same courtesy to you. However, if anyone sees anyone else about to fall off a cliff, that person should speak up. But only then.

This rule has worked well in my family for more than twenty years. It keeps the criticism and hurt level very low, yet it allows for intervention when someone is really headed for trouble. Note that the rule goes both ways. They can speak up about you. Remember that when you are ninety-seven and those whipper-snappers want to take your car keys away.

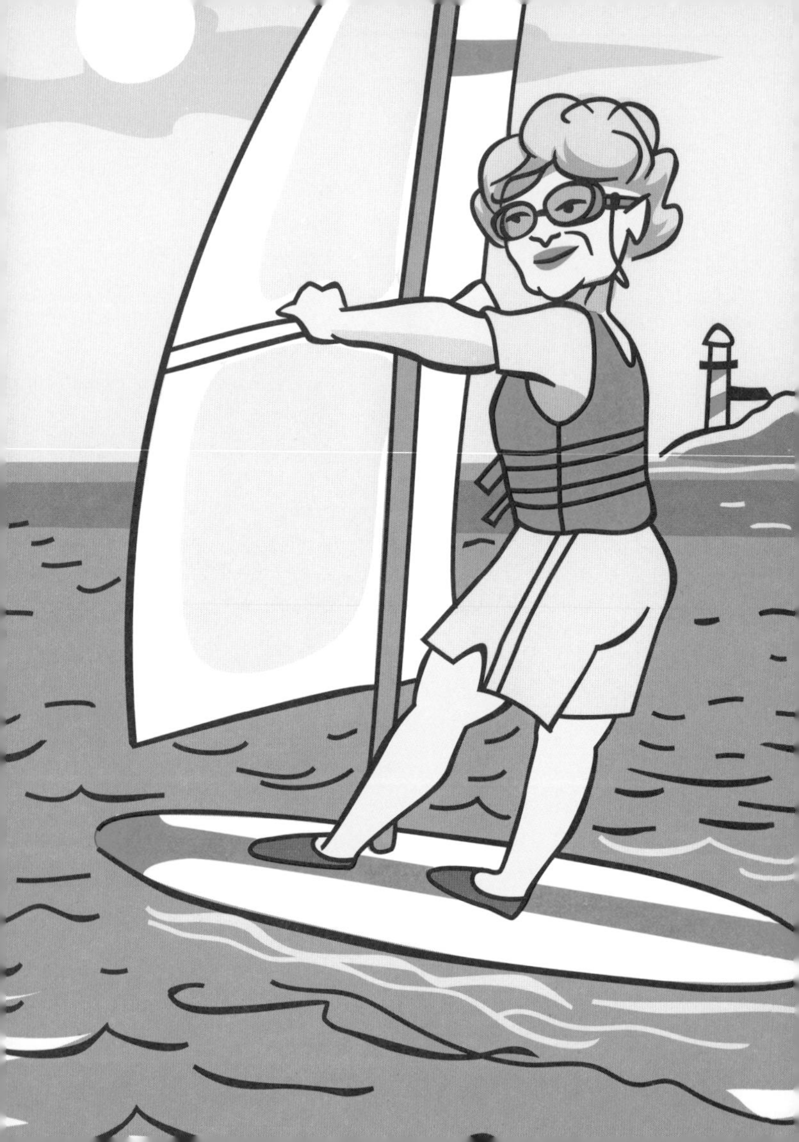

THE WORLD

Hot Granny Finds Her Passions

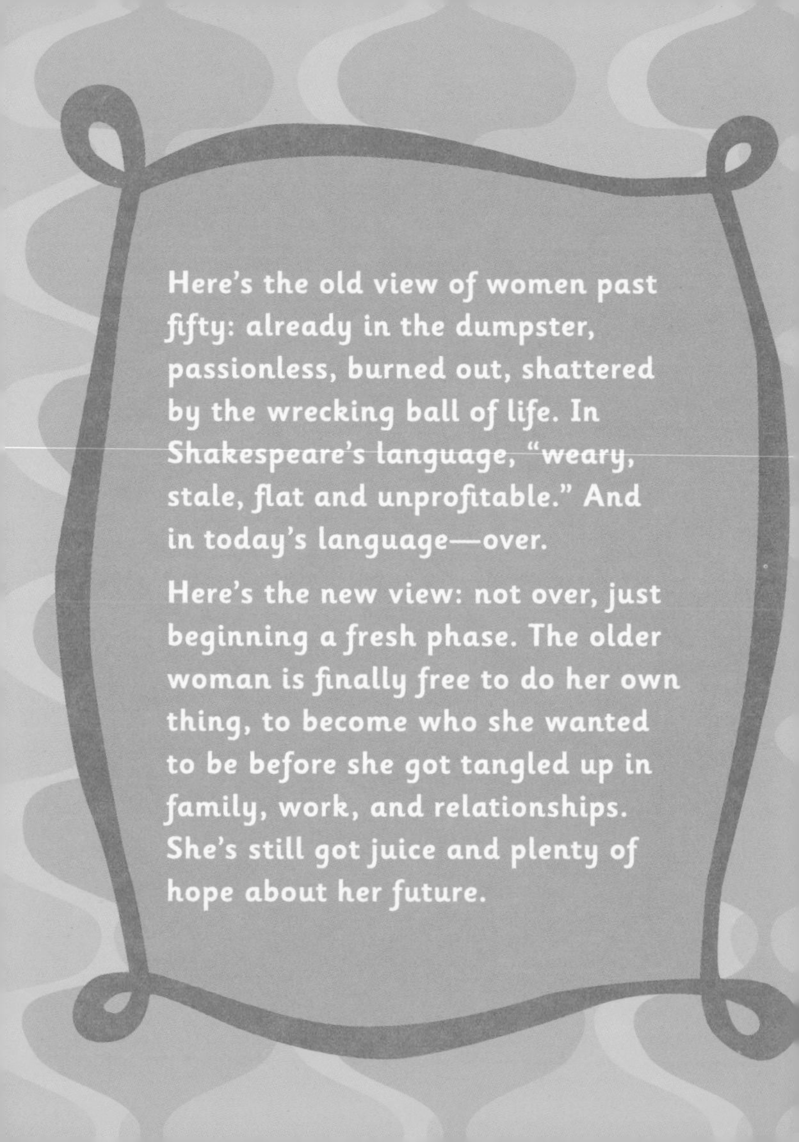

Here's the old view of women past fifty: already in the dumpster, passionless, burned out, shattered by the wrecking ball of life. In Shakespeare's language, "weary, stale, flat and unprofitable." And in today's language—over.

Here's the new view: not over, just beginning a fresh phase. The older woman is finally free to do her own thing, to become who she wanted to be before she got tangled up in family, work, and relationships. She's still got juice and plenty of hope about her future.

Me, I go with the new view. These are the years to dig your dreams out from under the debris that may have buried them by midlife. Think of your dreams as archaeological treasures waiting to be rediscovered.

But before digging for dreams, our minds should be clear of rubbish—specifically, the ageist stereotypes about what's possible or "normal" after fifty. Remember the 1970s, when we learned a lot about sexism and how it eroded women's expectations about themselves? Well, now it's ageism that we need to be alert to, a nasty packet of beliefs that can derail the older woman's hopes for her own future.

Consider some of the negative stereotypes: Older women are cranky, crazy, selfish, lonely, sad, messy, poor, dependent, sick, and incontinent. What's worse, they carry bad purses. Did I mention that they are also depressed, pill-popping, and useless? Some people even call us battle-axes, hags, witches, crones, and old bags—the last meaning the uterus is out of service.

Some of the stereotypes are but a vanilla version of the arsenic above. Grandmothers sit in rocking chairs and knit. They live to make cookies for their grandchildren. They are unfailingly sweet and will go gently to the next world, occupying only the heavenly real estate where the better class of angels lives.

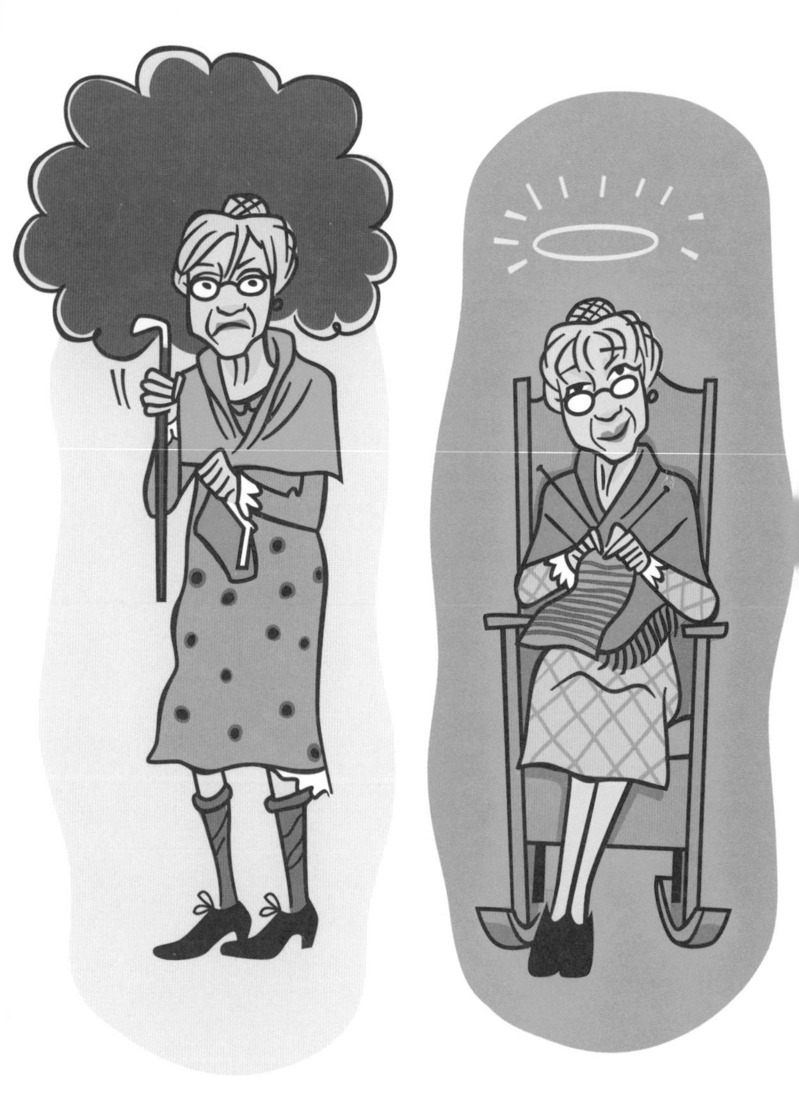

Well, either way, stereotypes are trouble. The trouble with negative stereotypes is that some older women come to believe them, and if they take these ideas to heart, they may end up with the self-esteem of a night crawler, afraid it's too late to chase their dreams. And the trouble with the "positive" stereotypes is that they confine women to a rocking chair and sainthood. And nothing is more exhausting than aiming for sainthood. Been there, done that. Gave it up. Good.

Finally, consider that no Hot Granny worth the title would allow herself to be poisoned by a stereotype. Instead, when you know that your older self is a worthy being, you are free to pursue the passions of later life, interests that may lead you to new friends and even to a mate.

Finding Passion

Today, the nonsexual passions of older women seem to fall into three main groups: a passion for making a difference, for helping others; a passion for creating, for expressing oneself; and a passion for traveling, for seeing the sights. Travel is covered in the next chapter, leaving us to consider here how a Hot Granny might make the world a better place and how she might express herself creatively.

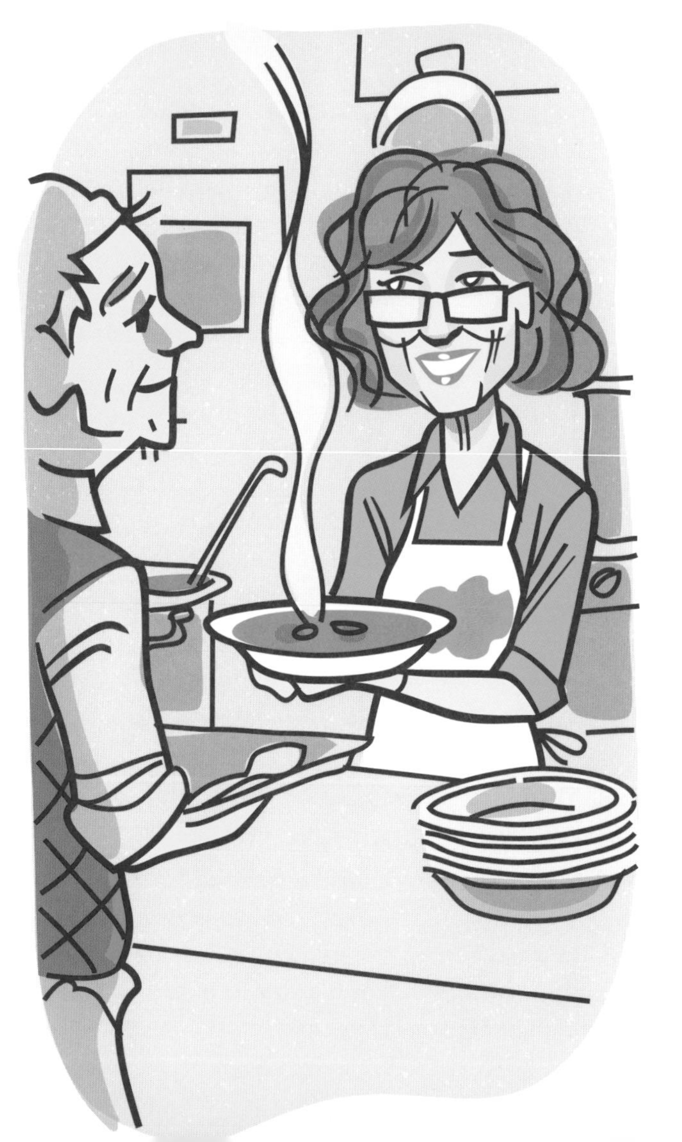

HELPING OTHERS

For some older women, finding a place in the world of philanthropy is a no-brainer. They know where they want to contribute their time and money, and so they do. But others of us may either be burned out with our usual do-good activities, or we may have retired to a new town.

So, we look around to see where we might fit in and what we might enjoy. Notice the word *enjoy*, for there is no point in saving the world by torturing yourself doing something you hate. In fact, begin by taking an inventory of what you love: animals, antiques, art, books and libraries, children, education, gardening, health organizations, history, music, nature, older people, politics, sports—all these and more will have volunteer opportunities connected to them. Check out www.volunteermatch.com.

Some Volunteer Opportunities

Gardener for a nonprofit organization · Docent at an art museum · **Helper on an archaeological dig** · Cook in a charity kitchen · Counselor at a hospice · **Usher at the symphony** · Crosswalk guard at the local school · Caterer for a fund-raiser · **Flower arranger at church** · Literacy teacher at a school · Receptionist at a hospital · **Hairdresser at a nursing home** · Judge at the county fair · Writer, editor, or photographer for a nonprofit newsletter · **Entertainer at a retirement community** · Driver for the disabled

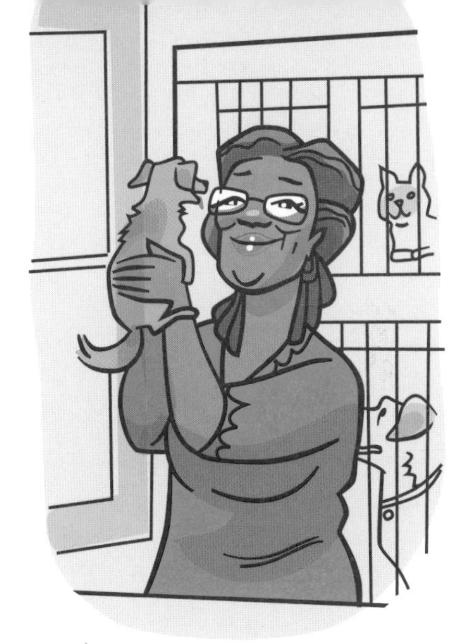

THE SMART VOLUNTEER

The trick is not only to get connected to the right place for your interests and talents, but also to do what you love within your chosen world. Example: Say you love animals, but the only open volunteer spot at the animal shelter is for a file-clerk position. You hate filing. So, don't do it. Don't fall into the compassion trap. Instead, tell the staff to call you when they have a way for you to work directly with the animals. Then move on to contact other animal-rescue organizations. Or consider providing home foster care for the shelter's overflow of animals.

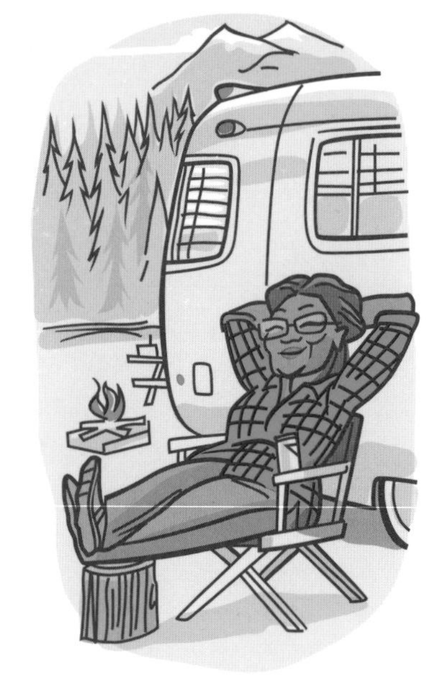

But don't chain yourself to a filing cabinet. There are some things we are too old for, and wasting our lifetime is one of them. Do what you love.

As for ferreting out good volunteer spots, many communities have local volunteer bureaus where you can look over the available positions, but talking to friends and keeping your antennae out for something that grabs your heart is also smart. And there may be ways to volunteer that you have never heard about or that are not listed at these bureaus. One of them is "workamping," a favorite with the many older couples who own a motor home.

Here's how it goes: federal and state parks often use older people as guides, greeters, and campground hosts, offering them free RV camping in a pleasant spot with water, electricity, and sewer hookups. In return, the parks will ask for maybe twenty hours a week of help. Pretty good deal. Win-win all around.

Workamping is a way to meet people from all parts of the world, and the lifestyle is especially suited to retired couples who both work at the park, have adventures together in their free time, and keep each other company at night. Check out www.workamper.com.

While finding a good fit for a volunteer job, note there are special opportunities for Hot Grannies who enjoy the grandmother role but whose grandkids may live a thousand miles away. For them, fostering grandkids is a good idea, and there are programs that will let them express their nurturing selves. One is the nationwide Foster Grandparents program. Look up www.seniorcorps.org, or call 800-677-1116 and ask for the location of the nearest Foster Grandparents program.

When volunteering, beware of the pitfalls of being kicked upstairs. You may love contact with the kids, the animals, the tourists, the patients—whomever you've chosen to help—but "they" may want to kick you upstairs to a volunteer position on the nonprofit's board of directors. If you love group experience like being on committees, making policy, and raising funds, do it. But if you just want to pet the puppy or tutor the kid, say "no" nicely, and stick with your passion.

Last, note that volunteer positions can lead to paid jobs. Hmm, doing good and getting paid for it—would that suit you, Hot Granny?

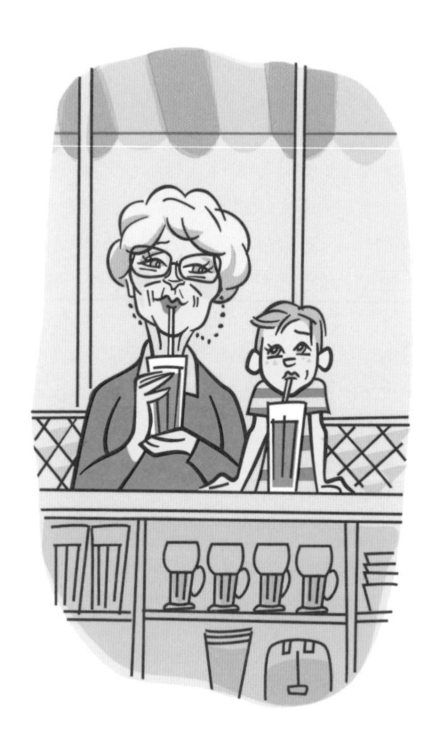

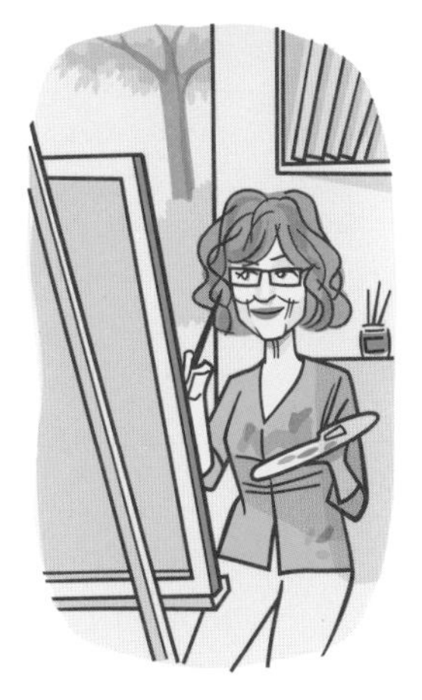

FINDING YOUR CREATIVE SELF

Of course, there are older women who know their own creativity and who have developed it over a lifetime. We see their work in galleries and wish we could do stuff like that. In fact, many of us arrive in later life still hoping that a creative self will some day announce itself to us—a muse descending through pink clouds to call on Hot Granny.

"Hey, here I am—your inner artist/photographer/writer/garden designer/quilter/potter/weaver/glass blower/jewelry maker/actress/musician/whatever."

Fat chance. Like expecting the perfect mate to announce himself.

No, Hot Granny has to put out a little effort to make either muse or mate appear in her life. You may have to try a lot of arts and crafts before you find one to suit, one that will engross your mind and spirit, add delight to your older years, and give you a deep sense of satisfaction. And it's not unrealistic to think you can make a new creative start later in life. Grandma Moses started her art career at seventy-five and painted about sixteen hundred works before her death at age one hundred and one.

Here's how to tell if you have found your creative calling: Time seems to flow by unnoticed when you are doing your work. When a Hot Granny's creativity is running in high gear, she is so absorbed that she does not look at her watch or realize that two hours have gone by. If this timelessness happens to you, bingo! You have found the G-spot of your creative life. But if you keep looking at your watch, then keep looking to find your creative home.

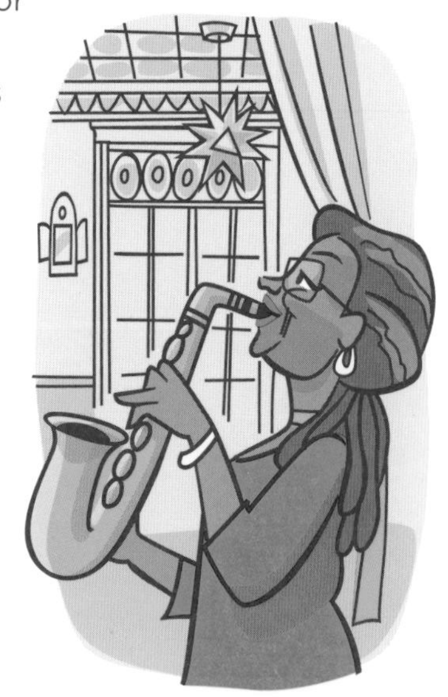

HOW TO FIND YOUR CREATIVE MATCH

Turn on your radar and look. Here are some places to explore.

Classes. Community college classes, university extension courses, classes at art centers or museums, courses at craft stores, classes given by artists at their homes or at an exotic spot, writing workshops at resorts such as Lake Tahoe or Maui, acting classes at local little theaters, classes available through Elderhostel, music lessons offered by players in local symphony or jazz groups. Community centers and senior centers also offer instruction in art and writing. Don't forget you can earn a degree or use classes to pursue the career you always dreamed about, whether it's being a jewelry designer or a master gardener.

Books and videos. There is a world of glorious how-to books and videos. Look in your library, bookstore, and online at www.amazon.com.

Retail stores. Look for stores that sell arts and crafts materials. Craft stores offer classes. So do stores that sell sewing machines and materials for knitting and embroidery. Read the bulletin boards at bookstores to see who is offering writing classes.

Online search engines. Go play at www.google.com. Enter the names of the arts that interest you. Add the words *instruction* or *class* for your area of interest.

Online instruction. An Internet search may lead you to the world of distance learning and Web classes—some from famous universities.

Artists. Last, look to artists and performers who are doing what you want to do. They often give classes to supplement their incomes.

GIVE IT TIME

When it comes to arts, crafts, writing, and performance, nobody begins as an expert. It's going to take a while to get on top of Hot Granny's artistic game. So, be tolerant of your beginning goofs and of your discontents as an intermediate. There's always something new to learn, always a way to improve, and some efforts will be clumsy.

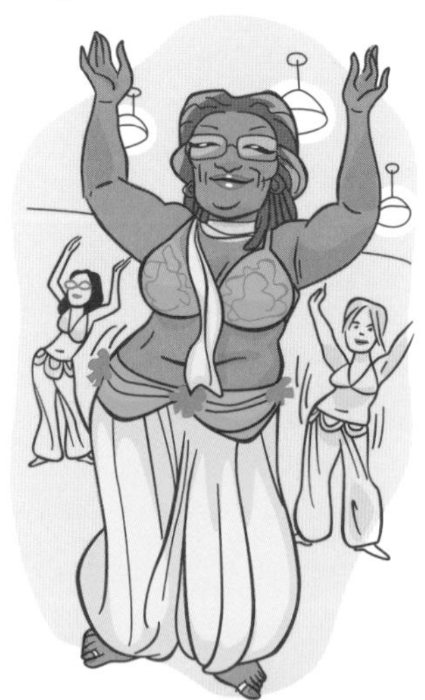

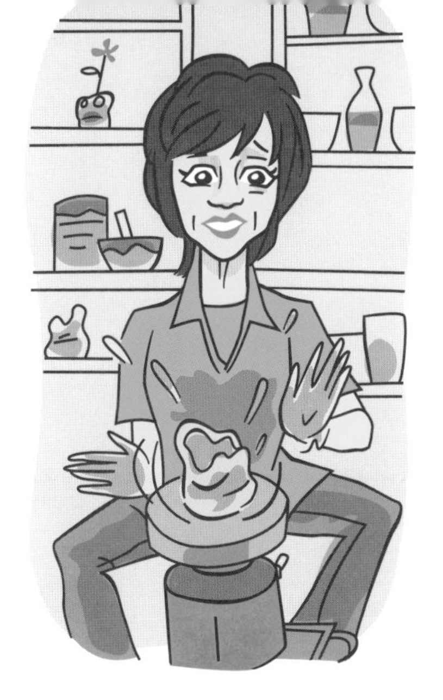

Progress, not perfection, is the realistic mantra here. Don't give up just because you are not Picasso by Tuesday. Neither was Picasso.

Last, discover the joy of being not so good. One of the secrets of happy living is to enjoy whatever you do, even though your performance is less than expert. Example: I was never more than an intermediate skier, and I had high times at that level. If you enjoy yourself, it doesn't matter if you don't win first prize with your chosen creative passion. A Hot Granny can have fun without chasing blue ribbons.

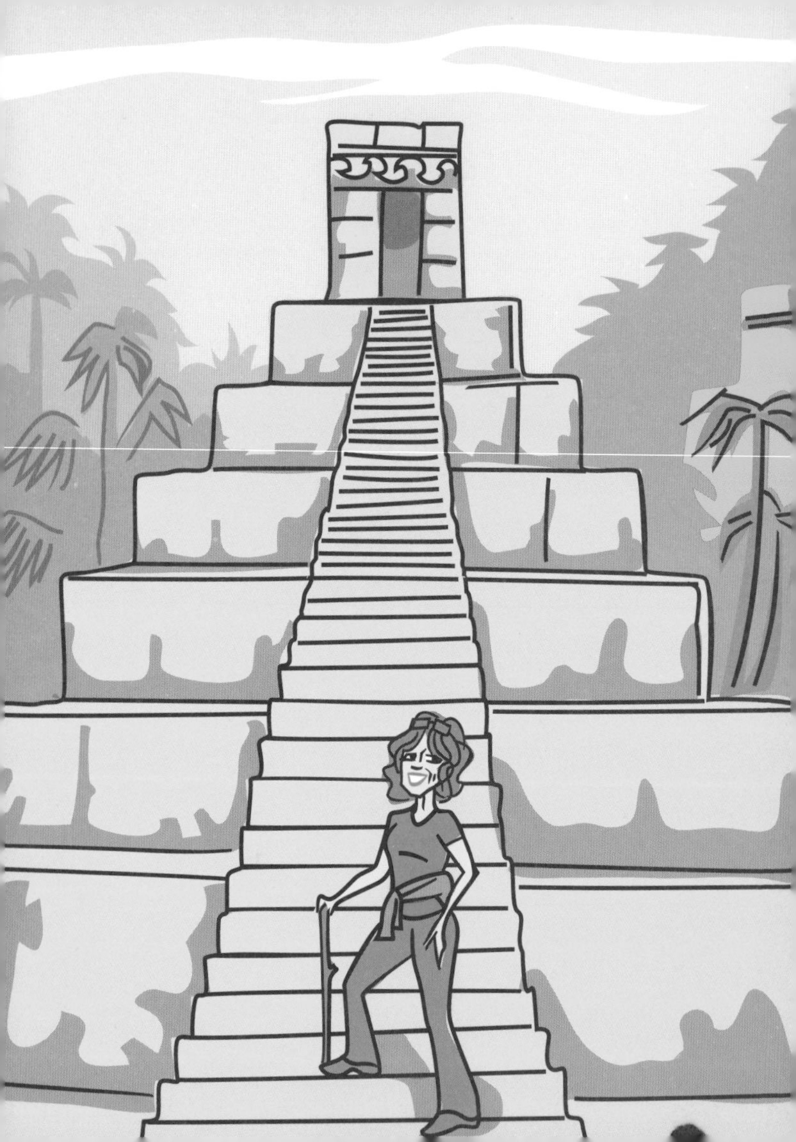

8

THE WORLD

Hot Granny's Dreams—Life Lists, Travel, and High Spirits

That darn biological clock. It never stops ticking. First it's the marriage clock, then the baby clock, and after the age of fifty, it's the mortality clock letting you know life is not forever. That clock has the loudest tick of all. Heck, it turns into an alarm with no snooze feature. It says: Wake up, woman. Life has limits.

Yes, we know that in theory we may die, and we secretly hope that an exception might be made for us—the world's first immortal Hot Granny—but when our parents pass on, the jig is up on denial. You have to know nothing is forever.

So what does a Hot Granny do with that knowledge? She has the time of her life.

Now.

Her motto is "Seize the day—carpe diem." Here are some ways to carpe your diems and yearums.

Life Lists

The first is to make a life list of everything you want to do, see, own, or experience before you graduate from the planet. It's a good way to make sure you don't miss out on what you really, really want to do in life.

Do not write this list on a sticky note, but get yourself a wonderful blank notebook and begin. Write down the basics, and then, as you think of them, fill out the specifics, and eventually cross out the ones that no longer make sense.

Check off the items as you do them, just like a shopping list. For it is a shopping list. You are shopping for what will fill the rest of your life with pleasure and the satisfaction that you didn't waste your time on the planet.

Here's an example of a life list.

- GO TO POSITANO AND DRINK WINE WITH A CUTE ITALIAN GUY.
- LEARN TO SAIL.
- GIVE A FABULOUS WEDDING FOR YOUR DAUGHTER/SON/SELF.
- TAKE A TRIP WITH YOUR MOM TO SEE THE OLD HOMETOWN.
- GO TO A CLASS REUNION.
- LOSE TWENTY POUNDS BEFORE THAT.
- ADOPT AN AIDS ORPHAN IN AFRICA.
- MAKE UP WITH YOUR SISTER.
- GO TO THE GALÁPAGOS (BUT FIRST FIND OUT WHERE THEY ARE).
- GET MARRIED (OR GET DIVORCED).
- RETIRE, AND READ EVERY BIOGRAPHY IN THE LOCAL LIBRARY.
- TAKE PIANO LESSONS.
- TAKE LINE-DANCE LESSONS.
- TRACE YOUR FAMILY HISTORY.
- SEE BRITISH COLUMBIA.

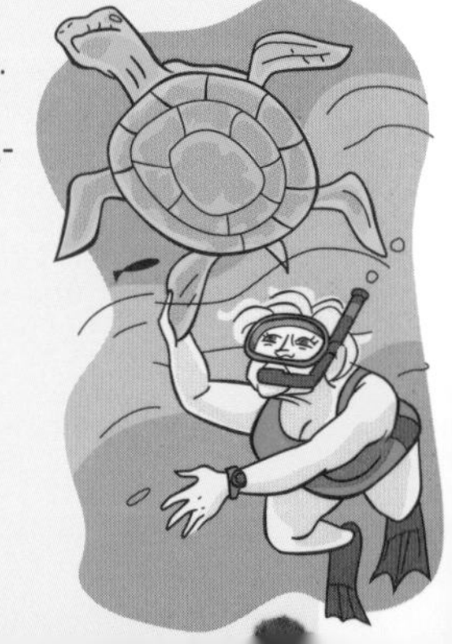

- BUILD A ROMANTIC GAZEBO IN THE BACKYARD.
- START A GARDEN OF OLD-FASHIONED ROSES.
- GET YOUR DAD TO RECORD SOME OF HIS CHILDHOOD MEMORIES.
- ORGANIZE AND FRAME THE GREAT FAMILY PHOTOS.
- LEARN TO PAINT.
- ONCE A YEAR, TRAVEL TO GOOD-MUSEUM CITIES WITH YOUR BEST FRIEND.
- GET A TAIL-WAGGER FROM THE POUND.
- LEAVE A GIFT TO YOUR FAVORITE NONPROFIT IN YOUR WILL.
- BUY A REALLY GOOD PAINTING FOR OVER THE FIREPLACE.
- HAVE LUNCH OUT EVERY DAY.
- TAKE A COOKING COURSE IN NAPA.
- LEARN FRENCH, AND TAKE YOUR NEW VOCABULARY TO PARIS.
- GET YOUR FAVORITE OLD SONGS—THE ONES YOU WORE OUT ON VINYL—ON CDS OR FROM THE WEB.
- MOVE TO THE COUNTRY.
- GET A PET LLAMA, AND WEAVE SCARVES FROM THE HAIR.

The trick is not to just write but to *do*. And if you hesitate to carry out your plans, ask yourself this: If you don't do these things in the near future, when will you?

If there are too many things on the list—I once had 109 on mine—then go through and pick the ones you would be really sorry to have missed if you were to expire tomorrow on the shelf of life. That will set your priorities straight. And remember that wishes can be downsized satisfactorily. I used to want a grand piano, but a little electronic keyboard satisfies the occasional Gershwin urges. And you may not have the money for a month in London in the summer, but you could fly over instead for a week in winter.

Travel

Travel is a promise that many of us made to ourselves when we were chained to our previous lives as moms, wives, and workers. Little time and money, plus other pressing priorities, kept many of us tethered close to home. But when a Hot Granny hits the age formerly known as retirement, she may finally have the time and freedom to hit the road. Sure, money may still be a problem—in fact, more of a problem now for those older women without pensions or investments—but there are ways for a Hot Granny to see the world without heavy expense.

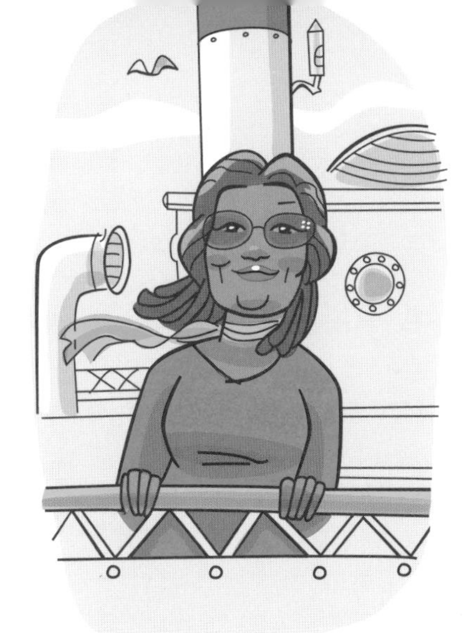

Do a home exchange. To avoid hotel and restaurant charges and enjoy the comforts of home while on vacation, trade houses. Yes, many intelligent people actually exchange homes with other intelligent people. They end up vacationing in a relaxed and private setting on the interesting turf of somebody else, and that somebody else may even live in another country. This may sound scary—trusting strangers with your stuff—but people who have traded houses are upbeat about the process. It seems to work because they get to know each other through e-mail, mail, and photos before they do the trade. Go to www.homeexchange.com to see how it works.

Rent a home or apartment. Again, the strategy here is to maximize your comfort and space, minimize your eating out, and stay someplace that is not corporately bland. To look over these offerings, go to Vacation Rental by Owners, www.vrbo.com. Also, look at www.craigslist.com under "housing, vacation rentals" for the town you're interested in.

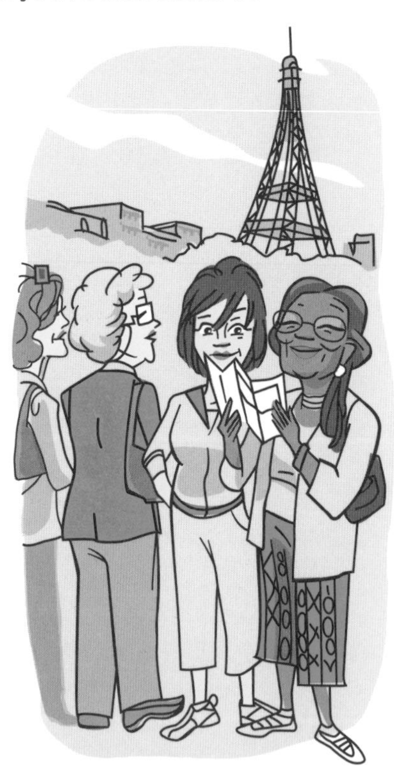

Go with a group. Split the costs and multiply the fun by asking family or friends to join in your expeditions.

Use budget travel sources. Check out the trips offered by organizations such as Elderhostel or by some of your local community groups. Call 877-426-8056 for an Elderhostel catalog. Also consult www.budgettravelonline.com.

Go off-season. The *Mona Lisa* will still be there in February, and there are worse things than Paris in the winter. Just add a long, warm coat; toasty boots; and a hat and gloves. You then have it made as a winter guest in the Northern Hemisphere.

Take your home with you. Go in a motor home. Make an investment in a good used RV, and use it as a traveling hotel for your later years. You can stay free or for perhaps $8 to $10 a night on public lands, such as national forests. Check out www.rvonline.com to see the range of motor homes. Leaf through the *National Forest Campground and Recreation Directory* to get yourself in the travel groove. Remember, Hot Granny can also use her motor home as a guest house. Motor homes are now tax-deductible.

Look close to home. Who of us has traveled enough on our own turf? Save the airfare, and see the sights around you.

Stay with family or friends. Don't overdo this, and do offer the return courtesy. It's rude to use others as a cheap hotel and may be hard on working families to accommodate a visitor for very long. The rule: If you are not likely to gracefully return the favor, do not impose.

Let the U.S. government be your host. The military owns some very inviting vacation turf that can be used by retired military personnel and their families. Think beaches and mountains. The offerings are vast and the prices reasonable. Check out *Military RV, Camping & Outdoor Recreation Around the World: Including Golf Courses and Marinas,* by William Crawford.

Look before you leap into your wallet. Don't make hotel reservations without checking out the experience of others. Look at www.tripadvisor.com for consumer rants and raves about hotels and restaurants around the world.

Use any available discounts. Discounts for older people seem to be disappearing when it comes to air travel, but there are all kinds of other discounts still available. Ask. A government discount may get Hot Granny her hotel room for half the stated rate.

Look at retreats for a quiet vacation. Though they are not well known as an option, there are thousands of abbeys, monasteries, and spiritual retreats where a Hot Granny can rest, relax, and recharge. These places

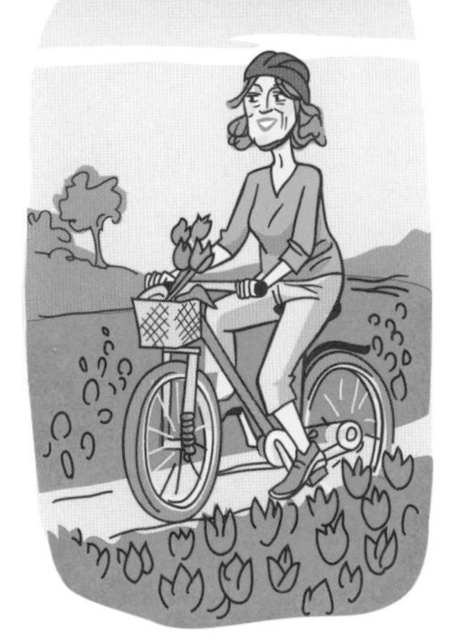

need the income from guests and, in return, can offer the public a shelter away from the mad, mad world. A Web search using the word *sanctuaries* will turn up more information.

Don't get sucked in by the extra fees of hotels. Hotels may advertise reasonable room rates, but their added fees can double your bill. Watch the fees for room service, Internet access, valet parking, $5 bottles of water, and such.

Go, even with a disability. Travel for the physically challenged is becoming easier. There is much information now on the Internet about accessibility and where and how to go. Look at this Web site, the proud property of a "disabled" man with a sense of humor: www.gimpon thego.com.

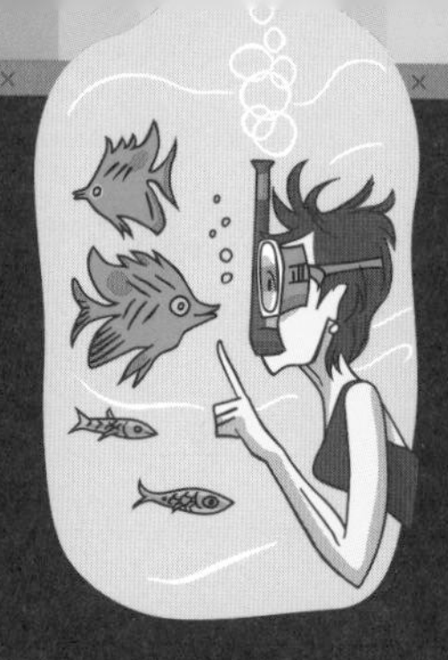

Where to Go?

A wine tour on a barge in Burgundy · A spring bicycle trip through the tulips in Holland · **A jaunt to see the old temples in Greece** · A hike in the New Zealand mountains · A trip to Vienna to hear the music · **A journey to the Chelsea Flower Show in London** · A snorkeling trip to Maui · A leaf-peeping weekend in Vermont some mellow October · **A visit to every national park** · A ride on a Washington state ferry to explore the San Juan Islands · A cross-country-skiing trip to the Sierra Nevada · **A gambling holiday in Monaco** · A body-surfing expedition off the San Diego coast · **A visit to the birthplace of a heroine**

And now, along with life lists and travel, there are still other ways for Hot Granny to maximize her joy in making it past the half-century mark. One is to pay attention to her morale.

High Spirits and Hot Granny

Few people talk about the state of their spirits, but everybody knows what it means to have high spirits or low spirits. I see it this way: It's as if each of us carries around a bucket of fresh, clear water. When things go well, when we are healthy, happy, and hanging out with people we like, our bucket overflows. But if we hit a rocky patch, spend time with negative people, or stay in bad situations, then the bucket gets a leak. Sometimes, during bad times, the bucket seems to go dry, with nothing but dust and spiderwebs at the bottom.

Now, our job as older women taking care of ourselves is to keep that bucket full and try to do the same for others. Full buckets all around—high spirits for all. Yes, mood building is important at all ages, but older people need to pay special attention to their morale.

Though later life can be great, it does have special challenges. Loved ones get sick and die, our own bodies can let us down, and our children have their own

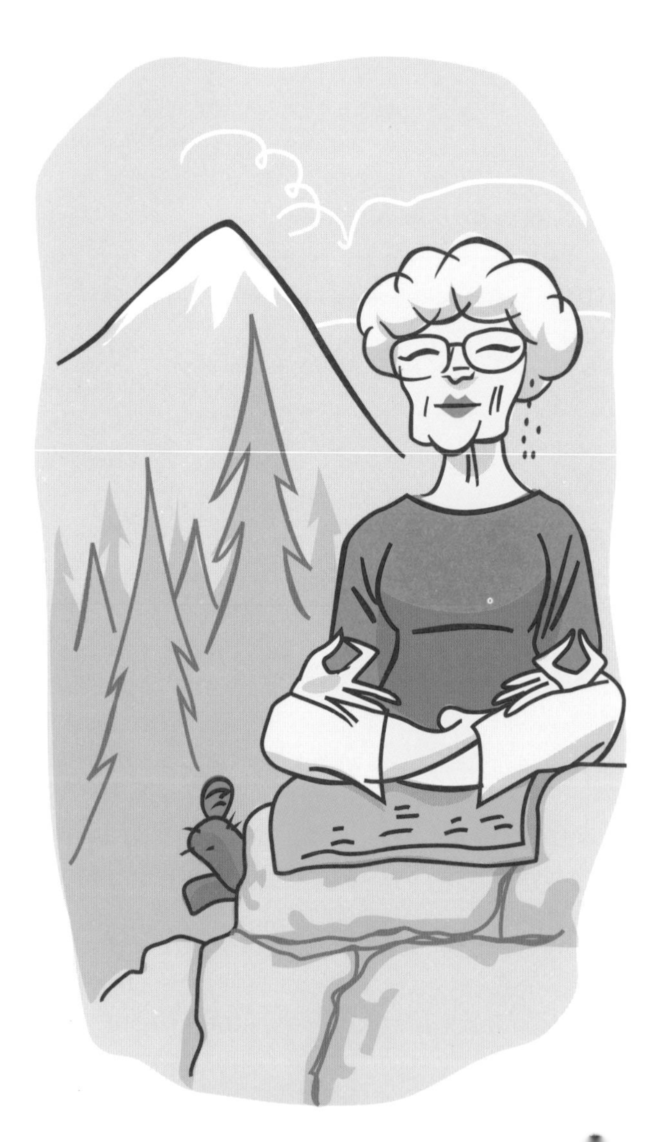

lives now. Their independence says that we were successful parents, but we are no longer needed and are left to hope we are wanted.

So, any Hot Granny who wants to seize her days and years should be taking care of her spirits and making sure that her bucket doesn't run dry. Here are some proven ideas.

Avoid negative people. Stay away from those who bring you down with constant complaints, criticism, and any other bad behavior. If they call or e-mail, you are busy. If they come over, excuse yourself. If you live with a person who's a major cramp, see a counselor. If you are a caregiver for a family member in need, get all the help you can. Look to the Family Caregiver Alliance, at www.caregiver.org.

Don't dwell on bad news. If you don't like how things are going in the world, write a letter, vote, or join a group to change things, but don't let the media drain your bucket.

Call friends. Think of friends as walking antidepressants.

Get outdoors. If you are in a bad mood, go for a walk. As Thoreau noted years ago, an outside ramble cures stale spirits.

Wear bright colors. The members of the Red Hat Society, women devoted to having fun, know the power

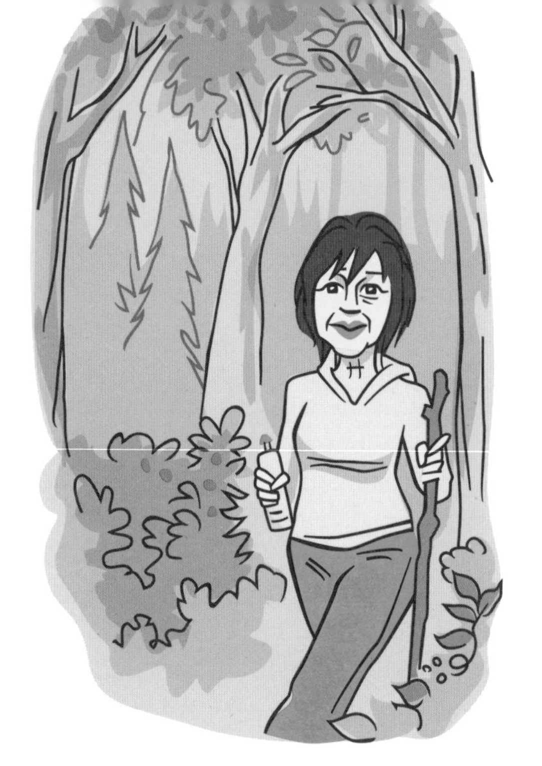

of color (see www.redhatsociety.com). So do the older women who like to wear purple. So did my mother—she who believed the answer to low morale was to put on lipstick, the Revlon solution to any dilemma.

Seek medical help. If you are depressed despite your best efforts to shake it, see a doctor. Antidepressants can work.

Get new buddies. Develop your social life, especially if friends have moved away in retirement or if you have relocated. Call someone who looks as if she has the makings of a Hot Granny.

Do something silly. Dance with your dog; sing old songs badly; wear a naughty T-shirt, if only to bed. Silliness is a mini-rebellion against convention, and a Hot Granny is a kind of rebel. She says no to the old way of thinking about the later life of women.

So then, to put this chapter in a nutshell: Make your plans on life lists, see what you want of the world, and keep your bucket full. That should do it in the enjoyment department.

Finally, as one aspiring Hot Granny to another, I have to say this: One of the great things about growing older is that we are finally the rulers of ourselves. Queen of the Kingdom, yes! When we were young, our parents and teachers were our bosses. Later, the supervisor, the client, and the mate had a lot to say about our lives, but by now we finally rule ourselves.

Some call this stage of life maturity. I call it Hot Granny's special time. After all, if the first fifty years were for other people, then we should have dibs on the next fifty. So stake your claim to the rest of your life, and enjoy!

When you find the time, please send me a postcard about your Hot Granny adventures or pass on your thoughts on Hot Grannyhood. I'll put the postcards up on my office wall to keep my bucket full.

MEL WALSH
P.O. BOX 478
CEDAR RIDGE, CA 95924

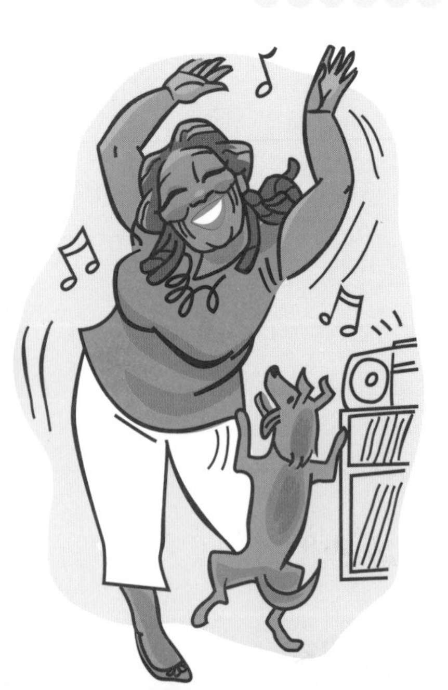

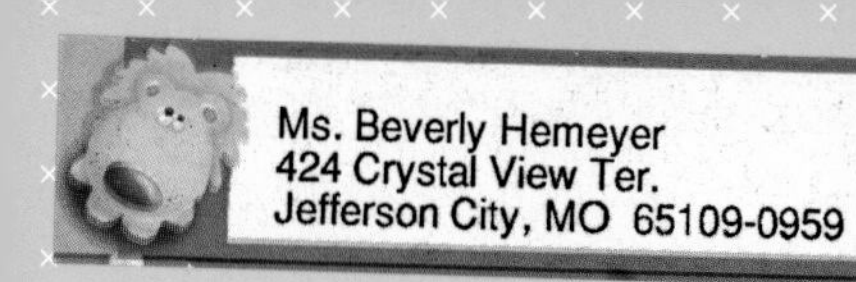
Ms. Beverly Hemeyer
424 Crystal View Ter.
Jefferson City, MO 65109-0959